Introduction

I'm no doctor, nor do I have any kind of degree related to the subject matter of this book. As such you are welcome to judge me accordingly but, a whole lot of people have changed the world and the way you live and they did not have degrees either. So I recommend you read this booklet first, before you judge me and I think you will see that a person does not need a degree to be smart, hard working, well informed, and indeed an expert in their field.

Although the horrendously overpriced rip-off colleges have not put me hundreds of thousands of dollars in debt, I am a consumer and I found myself looking down the massive vitamins and supplements aisle of a typical drug store and realized that there was absolutely no way a person could walk up, pick a multivitamin off the shelf, and get it right.

Furthermore, I realized that there was no way anyone could pick ANY product off of those shelves and get it right – that is, try to take something that would shore up what they perceive to be their weakness. And how could a person, like myself, even know what their weaknesses were in the first place?

This series of books intends to address this problem. I have done all of the research and I can tell you exactly which products have the best ingredients – which ones work – and where appropriate, which ones have such useless ingredients in them that they are worth avoiding.

I originally set out to augment Volume 1 "Dieting and Losing Weight" with a 2nd edition. But I have included so much new information that this book deserved to be added to the series and effectively replaces that first ever attempt to write a book for publication.

One in three Americans will die of cancer, and hundreds of thousands die each year from heart disease. These top 2 causes of death in the U.S. kill over 1.2 MILLION people accounting for 45% of ALL deaths each year in the U.S. and those numbers are on the rise.[167] Even with all of our amazing advances in medical science, things are getting worse, not better. And there is a reason for this: POOR DIET and LACK of EXERCISE.

Three things are killing people:
1. They eat POISON in the form of CANCER CAUSING ADDITIVES to their PROCESSED foods on a DAILY BASIS. (And they are exposed to other POISONS also on a daily basis, like DIESEL ENGINE FUMES, HARSH CLEANER FUMES, etc.)

2. POOR DIET: even if you eat right, most of the plants are being grown in dead soil that has been overused for decades, the only reason the plants grow at all is because of the massive amounts of fertilizers being used on them. Because of these conditions, many of the macro and micro-minerals and nutrients in plants are dramatically reduced, having been absorbed completely out of the soil by crops decades ago. Even the current crops, manage to eek out an existence based on their fertilizer sources of nutrients but cannot possibly be producing the supplements we expect from them in the quantities that they should, hence it is difficult to rely on the right foods because they simply no longer contain adequate levels of the nutrients that they should be providing us.

3. LACK OF EXERCISE: You cannot expect to be healthy if you do not engage in EXERCISE. I am certainly no expert in exercise but it is vital for OPTIMUM THRIVE-LEVEL health.

This series is designed to guide you through the bewildering maze of the essential nutrients and other supplements on the shelf at your favorite drug store and is not a substitute for professional advice. If you are currently on medication of any kind, you MUST CONSULT A DOCTOR before taking anything, including vitamins because they STRONGLY AFFECT the way your body works and could actually cause a VERY BAD REACTION in combination with certain strong medications.

Furthermore this series will show you how to eat properly, or rather, how to set up a regular food regimen that will provide you with all of the essential nutrients from natural whole foods rather than pills which have been shown in many studies to be far less effective than the whole foods they were extracted from or worse mimicked by synthetic replacements. More and more doctors and health professionals are starting to recommend natural whole foods over purified extracts and manufactured chemicals, a realization that I have been advocating for thirty years.

Think about this: hundreds of thousands die each year from heart disease and one of the chronic issues that can ultimately lead to this end is being overweight. And cardiovascular disease, like all other chronic health issues, does not kill out of the blue; it takes years, even decades to develop. If the average time span for a person to go from being a perfectly healthy adolescent, to having a life-threatening illness due to poor diet is 30 years, then right now as you read these words, over 18 MILLION people in the U.S. are on this downward spiral toward death due to cardiovascular disease aggravated by being overweight and this is, in most cases, PREVENTABLE. And no matter where you are along this path, you can always REVERSE COURSE and head back towards OPTIMUM THRIVE-LEVEL health and live a longer, healthier and happier life.

I don't practice holism or herbal medicine for two reasons. 1) When I give anyone a piece of advice, it is always basically a "trial and error" process, but many people are tempted to overindulge. If a little of something is good for them then they automatically figure that a lot of it must be extremely good for them and it never is. 2) It is an enormous responsibility to tell someone "Plant X will cure Ailment Y." Even if the plant has scientific studies showing this to be true, that does not mean that it will work for every individual on Earth. And giving someone that piece of information doesn't mean they will use the plant responsibly and correctly, and in many cases I would be relying on their ability to "self-diagnose" and they are not always correct as well as the fact that for serious issues they should visit their doctor first – not an herbalist.

Consequently, I generally avoid even casually mentioning the medicinal power of herbs to anybody. I do practice herbalism on myself and have so since my mother raised me on it, but if something goes wrong then I only hurt myself and have no one else to blame. However, by writing this book I am giving a lot of advice on medicinal herbs to a lot of folks and the potential for disaster is definitely higher than giving advice to friends because they know me and we can sit down and have a long discussion about their specific issue and I can cover safety in enough detail that they know the situation starting with the fact that I cannot take responsibility for the consequences of their decision to take my advice and I will not take responsibility if they misuse the remedy or if it does not work for them. Therefore, it is paramount that you understand the situation completely as well.

SAFETY WITH HERBALISM

Even the safest and most important substances needed by the human body like Oxygen and Water, can cause trouble in excess; hyperventilating will make you dizzy and drinking too much water can cause much more trouble than you might think. So even if these top two requirements of the body can cause trouble in excess then it stands to reason that EVERYTHING will cause trouble in excess. Even the most innocuous and healthy foods can cause serious issues through overindulgence and some Vitamins and all of the Minerals can become toxic in excess. As a result of this it is imperative that you understand the basic rules of safety regarding proper natural source nutrition and herbalism which are one and the same.

1) DO NOT "SELF-DIAGNOSE" – Quite often people can do this and get it right, but they are just as likely to get it WRONG. And that could have DEADLY consequences: something as simple as dizziness or ringing in the ears can be signs of a life-threatening health issue. Whenever you get some new symptom out-of-the-blue, you cannot afford to ignore it and you cannot afford to

3

ASSUME you know what is causing it. Even doctors go to other doctors to make absolutely certain they know what's wrong before they take up a course of action to correct the issue. If they feel that this is necessary and prudent – and they studied medicine for ten years – then all of us who have not studied medicine must seek a professional diagnosis as well. IF YOU HAVE ANY UNUSUAL SYMPTOM(S) GO TO A DOCTOR FOR A PROPER DIAGNOSIS.

2) DO NOT "SELF-MEDICATE" – Under normal circumstances, such as being overweight with no overt symptoms that could be warning signs of some serious health issue, you can certainly engage in the modification of your diet - convert to what doctor's call a "proper diet" and begin to exercise in order to pursue what I call "Optimum thrive-level" health. However, when it comes to serious issues such as high blood pressure, Type II diabetes, high cholesterol, etc, then the situation is different. By the time you experience symptoms of any of these issues, they may already be advanced to the point of being life-threatening. So following rule #1 – going to a doctor – comes Rule #2 – FOLLOW THE DOCTOR'S ADVICE. As long as your issue has not progressed to the point of being dangerous, you can certainly ask your doctor if it is possible to correct the situation with proper diet and exercise rather than take harsh prescription drugs. Most conscientious doctor's would sing and dance if a patient made this suggestion and was serious about making this commitment. But there are doctor's who might insist on setting you up for a lifetime addiction to prescription drugs because they are under a lot of pressure by the drug companies to sell them and they have a huge overhead; doctors are paying hundreds of thousands of dollars a year in malpractice insurance premiums and getting you hooked on harsh drugs gets you coming back for regular checkups and prescription refills, lab tests, etc. Most simple issues like high blood pressure and high cholesterol in particular do not necessarily need to be treated with drugs and all of this additional expense. The primary cause of two maladies is poor diet and they can be fixed by proper diet.

3) DO NOT OVERINDULGE – Everyone (including myself) is tempted to over-medicate. If one pill works alright, then two must work twice as well and ten must be an instant cure, right? WRONG. Always remember: MORE IS NEVER BETTER WHEN IT COMES TO STRONG MEDICINE. As a matter of fact, more is never better when it comes to ANYTHING your body requires no matter how simple and harmless it might seem. Even some medicinal herbs offered as supplements in pill form may not be necessary in the amount indicated on the bottle. In some cases this might indeed be the correct dosage for most people, but I am not most people – no one is. And we cannot ignore the fact that the manufacturer makes money by selling the item. So the faster you run out of it, the faster you will need to buy more of it.

4

4) BE CAREFUL OF ALLERGIC REACTIONS – I am surprised that no herbalist ever mentions this issue and it is IMPORTANT. In fact this is another reason I don't practice herbalism and it is the main reason I don't like herbal tea blends or custom formula mixes in dietary supplements. Whenever you decide to take a natural plant-based substance for the first time, the potential for an adverse allergic reaction is very real and possibly very dangerous – ANYONE COULD HAVE A DEADLY ALLERGIC REACTION TO ANY NEW FOREIGN SUBSTANCE INTRODUCED INTO THEIR BODY AT ANY AGE. Even if you have never had an allergic reaction to anything in your life, you could still have a reaction to any new foreign substance, even a synthetic medication and each natural whole plant contains HUNDREDS of chemical constituents and you could be allergic to any one of them. If you are going to try an herbal tea for the first time; MAKE A SMALL AMOUNT OF THE SUBSTANCE TO BE TESTED AND SCRATCH YOUR SKIN WITH A NEEDLE AND PUT A DROP ON THE SCRATCH. You do not have to draw blood with the scratch – that's too deep, and you don't need a scratch any longer than the droplet either. If it swells and turns red, then you know you are allergic to this plant and you need to try something else. You do not need to do this Schick Test for topical treatments like essential oils for external use only. For those, just place a drop on the tender spot of your inner wrist (below the palm of your hand) and watch for the same reaction (swelling, redness, itching, etc.) Supplement pills can also be tested in the same way. For gelcaps just squeeze the contents onto the scratch, for dry pills crush them in a mortar and pestle, add a few drops of water, mash this up thoroughly then apply to the scratch. Even those plants that do not cause an adverse reaction to the Schick Test could still cause a bad systemic reaction after being consumed. Always try a small amount of herbal tea (no more than a tablespoon) or a single supplement gelcap or half a dry pill. Have a contingency plan if you do end up having a severe reaction. (Have someone available to give you a ride to the hospital and take the product packaging with you so the doctor knows the cause and can determine the best treatment.) NEVER TRY MORE THAN ONE NEW SUBSTANCE AT A TIME AND TRY THEM IN SMALL AMOUNTS. Give any new substance, be it an edible plant, herbal tea, or dietary supplement at least two days before adding anything else so you are sure that it is safe.

5) ALWAYS GET A SECOND OPINION – I always verify the alleged benefits of any plant, edible or medicinal, from at least two independent sources. I list my own sources in the last chapter, but this advice pertains not only to a plant's nutritional or medicinal benefits but also its safety and to getting more than one opinion concerning your own nutritional or medicinal needs. If your doctor seems too eager prescribe drugs – especially for high blood pressure or high cholesterol, both of which can be controlled with proper diet and exercise – then ask another doctor. While I make every effort to verify the information I provide, typographical errors, omissions of critical details, and outright erroneous details are bound to happen not only in my sources, but in my own books as well, especially since I am not submitting these works to an editor. You have been warned: ALWAYS VERIFY ANY INFORMATION FROM ANY SOURCE ABOUT ANY SUBSTANCE YOU PLAN TO PUT INTO YOUR BODY AND SEEK A SECOND OPINION CONCERNING YOUR OWN SPECIFIC AND POSSIBLY UNIQUE SITUATION.

6) NEVER MIX DRUGS – Most people don't realize that all plants contain hundreds of identified compounds each and some of those compounds are very potent. IF YOU ARE CURRENTLY ON ANY PRESCRIPTION DRUG YOU MUST NOT TAKE ANY HOLISTIC HERB UNTIL YOU CHECK WITH YOUR DOCTOR. The harsh drugs prescribed for depression and many other drugs may be MAOI's (Monoamine Oxidase Inhibitors.) The problem is that Grapefruit also contains MAOI's which is why people on certain medications are warned to avoid this simple common fruit. As such if you are currently on ANY medication you MUST check with your doctor before adding any new plant to your diet or supplement intake. The vast majority of holistic plants, edible or medicinal, do not have adverse reactions in combinations because they are not concentrated like prescription drugs but, there are exceptions to this generally accepted rule like Coleus. The active compound, Forskolin, is very potent medicine (it is a strong immune stimulant) and people in generally good health should take it very sparingly regardless of any other natural whole foods or holistic herbs they might be taking. However, I do believe in the "Shotgun effect." That is, rather than depend on one remedy to treat a given issue, use many different remedies but not all at once. In other words, if you want to improve your immune system, take Coleus one day, Cat's Claw the next day, Astragalus the next, Eleuthero the next, and so on. By taking a different plant each day, you are ensuring that you get many different powerful phytonutrients, all of which promote increased immune system function in different ways which add up to make the immune system even stronger than any one holistic herb could. And at the same time you are avoiding overindulgence in any one of them and also helping to avoid MIXING them all at once which could have an adverse reaction. It's not ideal though because many phytonutrients are steroids which simply means that they act like hormones: they trigger our cells to begin behaving in a different way. Rather than actively participate directly toward some desired effect, they tell our own cells to start producing the desired effect. So these can have long-lasting and potent effects and these can have adverse reactions over the long-term. This is why I never recommend remedial plants to be taken daily or over long periods of time. The ultimate goal is to be healthy which starts with proper diet which this book will discuss in detail. Beyond that, you must endeavor to always consume the greatest variety of foods possible from one day to the next. This ensures that you will be exposed to the greatest selection of phytochemicals found in those foods, many of which may eventually turn out to be just as essential as those that have already been identified (the "Big 43" essential nutrients.) Since the goal is OPTIMUM THRIVE-LEVEL health and wellness, IF AT ANY TIME YOU FEEL WRONG OR A DISTINCT NOTICEABLE SYMPTOM, especially when you never had such an issue before trying these foods and holistic herbs, then the best response is to, STOP ALL NEW FOODS AND OTHER MEDICINAL HERBS IMMEDIATELY AND SEE YOUR DOCTOR.

7) WORK WITH YOUR DOCTOR – It may be necessary to find an open-minded doctor who is much more knowledgeable about the holistic herbs. Many doctors are beginning to embrace these plants because they are a subcategory of the Natural Whole Food Diet which they have all been recommending since the 1970's when people began eating more processed and packaged foods laced with CANCER CAUSING CHEMICALS than natural whole foods. But there are still many doctors who are unfamiliar with medicinal plants and very skeptical of their efficacy and safety and they will obviously always oppose anything you might wish to try. Far be it from me to suggest that the doctors are wrong, all I am saying is that no doctor would ever suggest that your diet should consist solely of Twinkies (completely synthetic food) and they cannot deny that the vast majority of all prescription drugs were discovered in plants first (salicylic acid or "Aspirin" was discovered in Willow Bark Tea used by Native Americans for aches and pains.) If you have been diagnosed with any serious condition such as kidney disease, liver disease, cancer, etc, you must FOLLOW YOUR DOCTOR'S ADVICE AND TREATMENT. The "Natural Whole Foods and Holistic Herbs Diet" is intended to take you away from a poor diet and toward a superior healthy and nutritious one and TO AUGMENT YOUR DOCTOR'S ADVICE AND TREATMENT BUT NEVER TO REPLACE OR SUPERCEDE THOSE EFFORTS.

One last important statement: Although I do list many "Top Recommended Supplements" throughout the book:

> I DO NOT ENDORSE ANY PRODUCT. THE PRODUCTS LISTED ARE THE BEST I CAN FIND BASED SOLELY ON THE MANUFACTURER'S OWN DESCRIPTIONS WHICH COULD BE MISLEADING.

Most manufacturers are honest and reputable and make every effort to provide a quality product, but "most" is not "all." If you have doubts check the Better Business Bureau and search for independent reviews of the products.

A good rule of thumb is: if it comes in a plastic bag or cardboard box then it is loaded with MAN-MADE CHEMICALS; specifically: artificial colors, flavors and preservatives as well as artificial sweeteners and far too many of these SYNTHETIC compounds have already been proven in numerous studies to CAUSE CANCER.

While some of these "foods" contain NOTHING THAT WAS EVER ALIVE, even those that are based on real plant and animal products are so processed and overcooked that most of their nutritional content has been processed out and cooked away.

I have found a few packaged foods that actually have no chemical additives in them, but they are indeed few and far between. You cannot go wrong if all you buy to eat comes from the fresh produce and meat sections of you favorite grocery store. One of the main criticisms I run into a lot concerning the Natural Whole Foods and Holistic Herbs Diet is: "Produce is saturated with pesticides and fungicides anyway." And while this is true, then the bottom line is that ALL foods – unless you grow your own which I HIGHLY recommend – are tainted with CANCER-CAUSING chemicals. So the only thing left to compare is the NUTRITIONAL value of the foods. Since most packaged and processed foods have had most of their nutritional content removed during the processing or cooked away, then the natural whole foods are the clear winners with respect to nutritional content. A fresh, white fleshed whole Red Delicious Apple with skin has an ORAC – Oxygen Radical Absorption Capacity, a measure of its antioxidant power – of 4275. In comparison, orange carrots (they do come in every color of the rainbow) have a score of 697. The point is that the antioxidants definitely help the body fight and resist CHEMICAL TOXINS meaning the fresh apple can actually help your body cope with the pesticides on it, but the packaged Apple Pie pumped full of preservatives like BHT has an ORAC score of just 190; no help for your body to deal with that proven CANCER causing POISON. [34]

Every molecule you eat goes straight to the Liver, through what the health professionals call affectionately, the HEPATIC PORTAL VEIN. Basically all of the capillaries in the walls of your intestines, that are absorbing every molecule of what you eat, gather back together into a big vein that feeds directly into your liver. This organ gets the first look at what you had for dinner, every time. This is how what you had for dinner gets processed into suitable forms to be released into the blood and how all of those molecules get regulated. Otherwise you would have dinner, say a steak and a potato, and the potato would be converted into sugars which would hit your bloodstream within half an hour and you'd be on the same sugar rush as if you had bolted down a two liter bottle of soda – that would not be a very good plan, and so that's why everything funnels into the liver. (Potatoes actually have a very high Glycemic Index, by the way; their starches do get broken down into simple sugars in the digestive tract and it does hit your bloodstream as if you chugged a two liter soda pop.)

The liver will grab up everything and then try to slowly release it back into the bloodstream over the next several hours, at least. The liver recognizes a vast number of "good" naturally occurring molecules in natural foods and if it does not recognize the molecules – i.e. they are MAN-MADE – then it treats them like a TOXIN and tries to permanently take them out of circulation. You can bet it regulates the electrolytes since a particularly salty meal would likely cause you to have a heart attack if it didn't (the electrolytes are involved in the electrical field of the entire human body and dramatically affect the heart which does have a natural pacemaker nerve clump.) And you can bet it does everything it can, including letting its own cells DIE for the cause, in trying to remove POISONS from the blood stream coming from the intestines.

Now the liver can take some abuse along these lines and regenerate on its own, that is its job, but pushing it to its limits and beyond every day leads to liver disease, liver failure, cirrhosis of the liver: too many cells have been killed repeatedly to the point where the organ is scarred and it can't grow past scars as it is being destroyed by the POISON known as ETHANOL – usually – and so the liver literally dies a long slow horrible death and takes the overindulgent fool through a similar long, slow and horrible death along with it. Yes, ETHANOL, the alcohol in alcoholic beverages is one of the worst POISONS you can pickle your liver in – while 4 ounces of alcoholic beverages like wine (13% or less) in one sitting one time per day is considered to be a maximum for healthy individuals it is still converted into ethanaldehyde which KILLS LIVER CELLS. Grape juice has many of the phytonutrients found in wine and Red Wine Vinegar is FAR BETTER FOR YOU and contains ALL of the phytonutrients found in wine.

Now let's look at a few food label ingredient items. I won't mention the actual food products I found these in, but suffice it to say that those "foods" are nothing more than beautifully packaged POISONS. Here are some of my favorite HORRORS that I have found in common "food" products:

1) SODIUM BENZOATE – This may be in every single packaged food product on Earth, or at least in the United States, as a "preservative." Well, it might keep the food the same color and texture for a longer period of time, but it is certainly not preserving the person who eats it. Case in point: Benzene, (the Benzoate ion simply has an oxygen atom bonded to it, which might help lessen its TOXICITY but it certainly does not make it into manna from heaven either) used to be found in every high school chemistry lab

in the United States, including my own many years ago. But you won't find it there any more. Why? Because a study found that the vapors (it is highly volatile with a unique aroma, another such small organic molecule with a strange unique aroma is Napthalene or moth balls) and those fumes are extremely carcinogenic and we can't have the children being exposed to them can we? Absolutely not! But apparently it is OK to make sure they get their daily DOSE OF THE POISON in every packaged and processed food THEY EAT EVERY SINGLE DAY! Even if Sodium Benzoate's ion is 1/10,000[th] the carcinogen as the precursor Benzene, the fact is that every man, woman and child in the United States eats this POISON almost on a DAILY BASIS. And the last time I checked 350 million divided by ten thousand is still 35,000; as in cases of CANCER. I don't want to be one of them, do you?

2) SODIUM CASEINATE – This is one of my favorites. Ever hear of Casein paint? Basically this food product had wall paint in it and the manufacturer had the audacity explain why this ingredient was in the food: "added for texture." They added this garbage – house paint – to give the food the right TEXTURE? Personally, I think I stopped wanting to eat paint by the time I reached the age of two years old, but thanks anyway.

3) SODIUM STEARATE – Another favorite, this is SOAP. Now I admit I've got quite the potty mouth, but my mother never washed my mouth out with soap, and as an adult I am not about to start either. These monsters didn't even have the decency to explain why they put the soap into the food either. Well I guess it keeps it clean right? Ever wonder why soap cleans so well? It bonds with fats and oils and is also soluble in water, this means that it grabs up the oils and dissolves with them into the water and then rinses away squeaky clean. Well I don't want all of my cells which are water wrapped in little bags of protein and OIL to get rinsed away leaving my bones squeaky clean … I'd like to keep all of my cells right there where they are! This stuff is appearing on the rise in vitamin pills as Magnesium Stearate. It is almost impossible to find a pill that does NOT have it. Personally, I don't want to swallow a small chunk of soap, but it looks like they are giving us little choice in the matter.

4) YELLOW #5 – This is a particular pet peeve of mine. This well known carcinogen – and I mean there are a multitude of studies showing this garbage to be a verified CANCER CAUSING KILLER – is in almost as many things as that confounded menace Sodium Benzoate. This garbage causes cancer. Do not eat any food containing it and the manufacturers will eventually get the idea and stop using it. Two major culprits that I have found are pickles and mustard.

5) The six major SUGAR SUBSTITUTES – acesulfame potassium, aspartame, neotame, sacharrin, sucralose, and sorbitol. I cannot speak for all of them but I can speak for some of them in particular.

Saccharin is a verified CANCER CAUSING POISON; in fact it makes an excellent cockroach killer. I found a roach dead in the powder, it couldn't even walk away – that's how fast the saccharin killed it. Personally, anything that can kill a roach is nothing I want to be eating, these are the only critters that survived the world's first thermonuclear bomb test, but they can't survive Saccharin. Aspartame also has some studies linking it to cancer. I think you're getting the idea: I'd rather risk rotting my teeth than dying of cancer. Now I know the diabetics are in trouble, they can't just go back to sugar. But that's ok; there are natural sugar substitutes like Stevia. As for the rest of us, do not bother consuming any artificial sweeteners, they cause cancer, period.

I understand that casein is a constituent of milk. Sodium caseinate is that ingredient likely reacted with sodium hydroxide (lye) to produce sodium caseinate. The problem is that any time a naturally occurring constituent in our food is CONVERTED from its NATURAL form into another compound, an ARTIFICIAL and UNNATURAL compound; it is also converted from a USEFUL and HARMLESS constituent in food into a USELESS and HARMFUL one.

Native Americans used willow bark tea for aches and pains. The pharmaceutical companies looked into it and discovered the "active ingredient" in that tea: salicylic acid. They learned how to synthesize it and produce pills of it and it works, but they have isolated a single constituent from the willow bark and sell it in a concentrated form: Aspirin. This is like listening to a single blaring trumpet while the tea is a complete orchestra playing a song. In other words, while the pill is the active ingredient and it does work, it also tends to punch holes in your stomach while willow bark tea does not. Even a natural ingredient isolated from the natural source and given in a pure concentrated form can transform the ingredient from a useful and harmless compound into a USELESS and HARMFUL one.

Now that you have several examples of additives to your food, what do they all have in common? They sound like they belong on the shelf of a college chemistry laboratory and NOT IN YOUR FOOD. And if it sounds like that's the way it should be, then the chances are good that YOU'RE RIGHT. So read the label and if it contains some SODIUM blahblahblahATE or blahblahblahIUM blahATE in it – then DON'T EAT IT!

If the food product has an ingredients label, and is inside of a cardboard or plastic wrapped package then it almost always has at least one of these manmade CHEMICALS in it, and if man made it, it is much of more likely to be POISONOUS, than if nature made it – even the same "exact" molecule and I'll tell you why right now.

No human being has ever SEEN an atom. There is evidence that they exist and I am not trying to deny that, what I am saying is that no one has ever gotten all the way down there to get a really good close up look at one. As such, there may be tiny differences between one atom and another, in fact quantum theory confirms that, and there may be extremely subtle differences between two allegedly identical molecules, one made in a lab and the other made in a tree. There is scientific proof for this statement as well: sugar. You have heard of "left-handed" sugar. It means that the molecule is large and extended in three dimensions like a shoe, it has length, width and height and a recognizable top side and bottom side and a characteristic, like the top view shape or bend in the shoe that makes the left one unique from the right one. And you can't just turn it over and use it, because your foot can't go through the bottom of the shoe in order to put it on, in other words, the left shoe and the right shoe are unique and can't be switched, you will never want to buy a pair of shoes in which there were two left shoes in it, unless you actually have two left feet, of course. The same is true of the three dimensional shape of the sugar molecule and interestingly enough, all plants make "right handed" sugar and they do not manufacture any left handed sugar. And in a laboratory, starting with say, carbon dioxide, and water (just like the plants do) humans could manufacture sugar, but without a "differentiating enzyme" they would make 50% right handed sugar and 50% left handed sugar. The differentiating enzyme would be any substance used in the process of making the sugar that itself has only right handed molecules in it, that could then control the outcome and make all of the resultant molecules left or right handed.

One more statement concerning that: since we can't make exclusively right or left handed molecules from scratch (starting with molecules that do not have left or right handedness to them) then that differentiating enzyme would have to be collected from a living thing, because life has been making exclusively right-handed molecules for eons. Suffice it to say that since WE are living things and therefore WE have a lot of exclusively left or right handed molecules in our construction and cellular processes, then it makes sense that at some point, if we encounter a quantity of the "wrong way" molecule, that it won't just be useless, but it might very well be POISONOUS to us as well. And there are such examples known to science; the right handed one is good for us and the left handed one is bad for us.

Now I have had a rather lengthy excursion into this subject of left and right handed molecules and chemists call any molecule that has a sufficiently complex three dimensional shape that it can have left and right handed molecules "stereoenantiomers" (YIKES! But now you've got yourself a nice $50 word to throw around at parties!) And now I can return to my original point; there is no way for us to know all of the subtleties within molecules containing even five atoms, let alone hundreds and many molecules involved in nutrition are huge. Tannins for example can contain over 3,000 carbon atoms per molecule. Therefore, artificial versions of any molecule are not necessarily the SAME EXACT MOLECULES and can therefore be subtly different in such a way that they are SETTING YOU UP FOR DEATH, likely in the form of CANCER, and at the very least are POTENTIALLY INEFFECTIVE in the case of MANUFACTURED VITAMINS: if man makes it then it is much more likely to be USELESS and/or HARMFUL.

So what should you buy? I'll side with the natural whole foods NOT POISONED ON PURPOSE WITH SODIUM BENZOATE, SACCHARIN, and YELLOW #5. I have found at least one food product that had ALL THREE of those in it. I am amazed that people don't fall to the floor, cold and hard, while partaking of that CANCER COCKTAIL.

No naturally occurring food will do you any more harm in moderation than those manufactured by some greedy profiteer. And natural whole foods usually have far more nutritional value than packaged and processed foods and that nutrition can help you resist the toxins found in virtually all modern foods. Fresh produce will certainly do far less harm than that little pink packet of cockroach killer in your coffee.

Check the labels. Some brands might add things you don't want. If the chicken looks too yellow, guess what they have bathed it in? Yellow #5, you got it! Incidentally when I indict that garbage I am referring to ALL artificial food colorings and flavors, not just that specific one. Don't eat that POISON.

Yes, I know that most artificial flavorings are chemically "identical" to the real ones found in nature, but why is it that artificial grape flavored things taste nothing like natural grapes? How identical are they? I believe I already warned you about this (sort of the same molecule not being exactly the same) and frankly I do not know how identical these molecules are to the natural ones, and I guarantee you that the greedy monsters POISONING YOUR FOOD with them don't know any more about it than the greatest physicists and chemists on Earth who would neither confirm nor deny my claims with anything more than quoting the Heisenberg Uncertainty principle, which supports my claim that they are different just as much as it would support their claim that undetectable differences are irrelevant. Sorry for the rant, but this stuff is KILLING US and if I get going down hill, there's no stopping me. The bad news is that the greedy monsters putting this TOXIC CANCER CAUSING GARBAGE into our food DON'T CARE EITHER: "Just shut up, BUY it and eat it."

READING THE NUTRITION LABEL

Back when the FDA made it law that all packaged foods had to carry a nutrition label, that label was far more extensive than the one they require nowadays. Most food manufacturers complained that the label was too large and therefore costly to print on their labeling especially for small items like candy wrappers, but the

TRUTH was that they didn't want the public to see rows and columns of ZEROS – that their "food" was about as nutritious as the wrapper and contained almost no vitamins or minerals and was loaded with tons of trash calories in the forms of saturated fats, trans fats, processed sugars (processed cane sugar and high fructose corn syrup both of which are DEADLY proven causes not just of Type II Diabetes but CANCER as well) and cholesterol.

So the FDA caved in to the demands of the greedy billionaire monsters and now only requires a smaller "more concise" nutrient label on packaged foods as a bare minimum requirement to comply with the law. And this label really only brings two useful pieces of information now: 1) How many calories are in a single serving and 2) What form of calories they are. What is now lacking is the complete listing of the vitamins and minerals and all that is left on this new abbreviated nutrition label is Vitamin A, Vitamin C, Calcium and Iron. There is no question that these four are indeed important and as a matter of fact most people do not get nearly enough of either calcium or iron from foods natural or processed on a daily basis and chronic deficiency of either (and likely both) can lead to terrible consequences like disease and dying before your time.

However, all of the other vitamins, minerals and essential nutrients are just as important and chronic deficiencies in them can be just as bad (disease and death) but now we can't check the label to see if the food is bringing enough things like Vitamin B5 – Pantothenic acid, or Chromium. Some nutrition labels embellish them and list extra nutrients if the food has a good amount of them in it, so we can take away from this: if the nutrient is not in the nutrient label listing, then it has little to none in it

THE TYPICAL NUTRITION LABEL

I have chosen as our typical sample nutrition label, the one included on the side of a typical box of "Macaroni and Cheese." This is a rather dreadful product for a number of reasons including the actual ingredients. I will skip that horror show here, but suffice it to say that it is loaded with chemicals and crud like processed wheat flour as well as that ubiquitous and apparently unstoppable bane: SOYBEAN by-products which are nothing but than CHEAP GARBAGE FILLERS. It takes up space and has weight and It is cheap which is why just about all packaged foods now have SOY in them, and many studies are now showing that this crud is BAD FOR HUMAN CONSUMPTION; in other words, it is TOXIC. I bet the people who wrote and produced the movie "Soylent Green" had no idea how prophetic it would turn out to be. (Thankfully, the manufacturers of our foods are not cooking PEOPLE into little green squares… yet!)

The formats of nutrition labels can be different and the one on the side of the slender box of "Mac and Cheese" that I am using is laid out differently than the way I shall present it here, but they all say the same things.

Nutrition Facts

Serving Size 2.5oz (70g/about 1/3 box)
Makes about 1 cup
Servings per Container about 3

Amount per Serving	Mix	Prepared
Calories	250	400
Calories from Fat	10	150

% Daily Value**		
Total Fat 1g*	**2%**	**26%**
Saturated Fat 0g	**0%**	15%
Trans Fat 0g		
Cholesterol 0mg	**0%**	**0%**
Sodium 580mg	**24%**	**31%**
Potassium 160mg	**5%**	**5%**
Total Carbohydrate 52g	**17%**	**18%**
Dietary Fiber 2g	**8%**	**8%**
Sugars 2g		
Protein 8g		

Vitamin A	0%	15%
Vitamin C	0%	0%
Calcium	2%	4%
Iron	10%	10%
Folic Acid	35%	35%

*Amount in mix. Prepared contributes an additional 150 calories (140 Calories from fat), 16g Total Fat (3g Saturated Fat, 3.5g Trans Fat), 160mg Sodium, 30mg Potassium, 1g Total Carbohydrate (1g Sugars), 1g Protein.
**Percent Daily Values are based on a 2,000 calories diet. Your daily values may be higher or lower depending on your calories needs:

Calories		2,000	2,500
Total Fat	Less than	65g	80g
Sat Fat	Less than	20g	25g
Cholesterol	Less than	300mg	300mg
Sodium	Less than	2400mg	2400mg
Potassium		3500mg	3500mg
Total Carbohydrate		300g	375g
Dietary Fiber		25g	30g

Calories per gram:
Fat 9 * Carbohydrate 4 * Protein 4

INTERPRETING THIS LABEL

At a glance the bottom third of this label is a description of the fact that the additives used in the preparation of the mix add a lot of

15

calories and fat: the additives to prepare this Mac and Cheese according to the package directions are 4 tablespoons of butter and ¼ cup of 2% skim milk. Any deviation from that will of course change these numbers.

Also of great interest is the fact that the FDA has CHANGED the RDA amounts of Sodium and Potassium from the numbers I have been using over the past ten years. The old values I have been using indicated a 100% RDA for Sodium of 2900mg and they have lowered this to 2400mg which is actually a HUGE amount (500mg less than before.) And the new 100% RDA of Potassium is set at 3500mg up from 3200mg. Both do play similar roles as electrolytes and both are necessary in the nerve-ending-to-muscle cell synapses. These numbers likely reflect the latest contributions from the studies in which excess Sodium has a confirmed affect of raising blood pressure while more Potassium tends to lower blood pressure.

1) Serving Size 2.5oz (70g/about 1/3 box) – This is a critical part of the nutrition label that most people either ignore or fail to "Do the Math" with it to see how many calories of the product they are actually eating at a given sitting. It's an important consideration with this product because the directions are for preparing the ENTIRE BOX (by adding those 4 tablespoons of butter and ¼ cup of 2% SKIM MILK) and nobody I know is going to try to measure out 1/3 of the box.

2) Servings per Container about 3 – This is the key piece of information in the header of the label. If you are consuming the whole container in one sitting then this tells you the MULTIPLIER for ALL of the values listed below and we will be multiplying everything by 3.

3) Amount per Serving… Mix… Prepared – These column headers point out the amount of the item and distinguish between the raw contents of the package and the contents prepared by FOLLOWING the DIRECTIONS and the AMOUNTS of the suggested ingredients to be added. Any deviation will change the values in the "Prepared" column possibly SIGNIFICANTLY.

I should point out that this particular food label has the added complication of the fact that it is a MIX and you must add other ingredients and that our choices of the amounts and kinds of ingredients that you add will change the numbers of the final product that you eat. Most products that are "Ready-to-Eat" do not have this second column of values and are thus much easier to read. I chose this label to give you a good example of one of the more complicated nutrition labels.

4) Calories… 250… 400 – Remember that they are using ONE serving for these numbers but we will use the entire box so we have to multiply EVERYTHING by 3: the WHOLE BOX contains 750 calories and prepared according to the directions will yield a pot of Mac and Cheese with a total content of 1200 calories.

5) Calories from Fat… 10… 150 – Clearly the MIX doesn't bring very much fat, but the butter and milk, whatever kinds and amounts you use, certainly will bring most of the fat in the final Mac and cheese that you sit down to eat: 30 calories in the WHOLE BOX (unprepared) and an estimated 450 calories from fat in the final cooked whole box. Since you can't eat it raw, you have no choice but to add butter and milk which will bring up the amount of fat in the final cooked product.

5) % Daily Value** – Now they will tell you what percent of each item this food will bring with the understanding that your daily total should be near no more than 100% for harmful items including Saturated Fat and Cholesterol. The double asterisk leads to a point underneath the lists which I will discuss when we get to it.

6) Total Fat 1g*… **2%… 26%** – This row points out again that the MIX itself is not bringing very much fat but the butter and the milk certainly will. The asterisk leads to an explanation of this further down in the food label which I will elaborate on when we get to it. Don't forget to multiply that 26% by 3 = 78%. This one item will give you over ¾ of our daily allowance of fat. So you better not eat any other food with fat in it for the rest of the day!

7) Saturated Fat… 0%… 15% – This unprepared product contains no saturated fat but because we must use butter and milk it forces us to introduce about 15% of our daily allowance PER SERVING so TIMES 3 = 45%, nearly half of what we should eat daily in this one item.

8) Trans Fat 0g – This has no RDA because it is ARTIFICIAL and TOXIC. Be glad this product has none in it but your ARTIFICIAL BUTTER could be LOADED WITH IT. And dumping 4 table spoons into the pot could be terrible for your HEART HEALTH.

9) Cholesterol 0g… 0%… 0% – While the product brings none, this assumes that BOTH the butter you have chosen and the milk that you have chosen do not contain any cholesterol which is not necessarily true. BOTH of my choices DO have cholesterol in them.

10) Sodium 580mg… 24%… 31% – This is exactly why the medical industry first went on its anti-salt crusade, because food manufacturers are DUMPING MASSIVE AMOUNTS of POOR QUALITY SALT into EVERYTHING they make. This product is OVERLOADED with it and the WHOLE BOX contains 72% of your daily requirement of Sodium by itself. Because of this you cannot use IODIZED SALT or SEA SALT to help get our IODINE because you have already loaded up on Sodium in this product. This is the #1 REASON NOT to eat packaged products like this unless they are LOW SODIUM VERSIONS (very difficult to find in cooking mix products, by the way.)

11) Potassium 160g… 5%… 5% – It would have been far better for us if the manufacturer had bothered to add a boat load of Potassium salt rather than plain GARBAGE Sodium salt, but they didn't obviously. Nevertheless we do need a lot of Potassium so this one is a welcome sight even though the WHOLE box will only provide you with 15% of the RDA for this important mineral.

12) Total Carbohydrate 52g... 17%... 18% – There is a trick to this one. They have already discussed the fats separately and two lines down they reveal the amount of sugars (a carbohydrate) as 2g (2 grams) while this line says 52g. So what are these other 50 grams of carbohydrates in this food? STARCH which is the very definition of TRASH CALORIES that no one should be eating. They come from the wheat flour in the macaroni pasta in the package. We DO need calories, but not a boat load of TRASH CALORIES. The best form of calories you can get from your foods is natural sugars (but not that processed white crystal GARBAGE) and UNREFINED POLYUNSATURATED fats (found in seeds and nuts which are high in essential nutrients and WORTH the calories in these forms) and SOME PROTEIN, but NO SATURATED FAT and NO STARCH. Multiply by 3 so this box is providing 51% of your DAILY CALORIC intake as STARCH.

13) Dietary Fiber 2g... 8%... 8% – Fiber comes from plants and it is the wheat flour in the pasta that is bringing all of this fiber. Fiber is good for you but the rest of the contents of this product make this food so bad that it isn't worth the few things that are actually good in it.

14) Protein 8g – This one needs a little explanation as well. First, there is no set RDA for protein in general although the FDA does recommend a minimum of 110g of Complete Protein (contains all nine essential amino acids) and this protein is coming from the pasta made from wheat and eggs. So we do not know how much of this is Complete Protein and the manufacturer is not obligated to tell us either. Expect most of it to be wheat protein (i.e. GLUTEN.) We also have to multiply by 3 so the box provides 24g of poor quality protein and down at the bottom they mention that there is roughly 4 calories in each gram of protein so this totals 96 calories from protein. We do not add it to the totals above, it is already included in those numbers.

15) Vitamin A... 0%... 15% – Finally, we have come to the part of the nutrition label that actually deals with NUTRITION! And the first item, Vitamin A, is ONLY coming from the milk that we provide and the entire box contains ZERO.

16) Vitamin C... 0%... 0% – Well, not even the milk helps with this critical nutrient. A TOTAL ZERO as far as Vitamin C goes. I can already think of a dozen side dishes for dinner that are FAR healthier than this nonsense: 4 oz of cabbage will provide less than 50 calories AND 100% RDA of Vitamin C.

17) Calcium... 2%... 4% – While there is a little calcium in both the package contents and the milk you provide, it will not be nearly enough to meet your daily requirements even though this product does bring a boat load of TRASH CALORIES which will prevent you from adding GOOD natural whole foods that WILL bring you the calcium you need.

18) Iron... 10%... 10% – The whole package will bring you 30% of your RDA for this critical nutrient, but where will you get the rest especially when this package cost you 1200 calories?

19) Folic Acid... 35%... 35% – Folates are very difficult to find and wheat, especially whole grain products and wheat germ are some of the best sources. Even though the whole box does provide you with just over 100% of this important vitamin, the cost in TRASH calories and Sodium doesn't justify it at all.

20) *Amount in mix. Prepared contributes an additional 150... – This line explains that all of the calories and fats are coming from the milk you provide and NOT their product.

21) **Percent Daily Values are based on a 2,000 calories diet... – This line and the rest of the label explains that the percentages are based on a diet of 2,000 calories per day and then they lay that out and compare it to a diet of 2,500 calories per day showing you the TOTALS of each type of nutrient that are recommended. It is all good information but let's be clear: we all know we need to stay away from: Sodium, Saturated Fat, and Cholesterol. The "recommended" amounts of these in the 2,000 calorie per day diet that they line up can be CONFUSING. It doesn't mean that you should eat those amounts it means these should be maximums and that you should try to stay BELOW those amounts as much as possible.

CONCLUSION

Now take a moment to consider the following: how long would you survive without air, in particular oxygen? A few minutes at most. We could therefore say correctly that gaseous oxygen is the ultimate and most essential of all nutrients. Without it a human body shuts down and dies within minutes. This is because the oxygen provides the "oxidizer" for our cells to burn fuel (sugars mostly) from which they derive the energy to function. No energy to function: no life, and the main organ that has by far the highest demand for oxygen is the brain and that's exactly why you die so fast without air, because your brain, properly functioning, is that which is conscious and is, in essence, you. It is fascinating to note that most of the rest of the body can get along quite well for extended periods of time without oxygen, but that is of no use when the brain, which is the person, dies so fast without it.

Now our respiration, our breathing which provides this most essential of all nutrients, only needs to take up oxygen (and get rid of built up carbon dioxide which is the result of the metabolic burning of the sugars in our cells) and nothing else; a very simple bodily function and requirement.

The point I am driving at here, is that although the process of eating is not as imperative as breathing, in that you will not starve to death in minutes if you stop; this does not change the fact that if you do stop eating, then you will die. Therefore eating is an imperative process, as imperative as breathing, even though the time delay between stopping it and dying is much more protracted, the outcome is the same.

But the major difference is that eating, which involves the consumption into the digestive tract of essential nutrients, is the opposite of the simplicity of breathing, in which we do it to take up one simple nutrient. In eating, we absorb gigantic collections of gigantic molecules in such profusions and complexities that we may never be able to fully analyze a complete and healthy natural diet consisting of fruits, vegetables, and animal products.

But although we may not be able to fully chemically analyze our nutritional needs, that does not mean that those needs do not exist and it does not mean that we should just throw our hands up and give up. All that this means is that the mad scientists will never be able to provide us with a George Jetson diet of nothing but manufactured pills that will provide OPTIMUM THRIVE-LEVEL health over a long lifespan.

What I ultimately want to convince you of, with this argument is that:

1. There can never be an adequate substitution for natural foods. You can certainly take a Vitamin A pill to make sure that you get enough each day, but carrots contain not only all the Vitamin A that you need, but it is in the form of beta-Carotene which is a powerful antioxidant that helps defend your entire body and all of its cells from being damaged by free radicals or "oxidants." But this exact same substance can be easily converted by the liver into more Vitamin A as needed: that's why I recommend to anyone concerned about Vitamin A to eat carrots, as many as you like, you very likely will not overdose on beta-Carotene although you certainly CAN overdose on pure Vitamin A.

2. By eating natural foods you will take in nutrients that no one even knows exist yet, but that the human body still needs. The more variety you have in your natural whole food diet, the more likely you will take in something that your body desperately needs.

3. Cravings have been suspected for years to involve a method by which the brain detects a serious deficiency, and the craving is the way in which the brain drives the person to get the missing nutrient. Listen to your cravings and more importantly, keep rotating and changing your diet from one day to the next so that you never fall short for more than five days in a row of anything your body might need.

4. We know that all of our food, especially in the developed countries, from the plants, fruits, vegetables, grains, to the livestock that feeds on these plants are seriously lacking in critical nutrients because of the long dead dirt in which they have been cultivated. But the grape still looks like a grape, so it

has still been able to construct its cells in all of their amazing complexity despite these shortcomings and therefore it has constructed complex molecules, that the mad scientists still have yet to discover or understand, and that your body needs in order to survive and to thrive. So despite my warnings that the plants and animals we eat are deficient, that does not mean that they are devoid of nutritional value. You must eat as many all-natural items in as much variety as you can in order to maintain optimal health and you must avoid ALL fake food; manufactured and processed foods, because they are rife with cancer causing poisons and the processing has destroyed most if not all of the potential nutrients in them as well.

5. By sticking to the Natural Whole Foods and Holistic Herbs Diet you won't have to check nutrition labels (and very few have them anyway) because the vast majority of them especially the plants are Net Negative Calorie foods: foods below 30 cal/oz. These are all far more nutritious than packaged and processed foods, lower calorie, and are therefore "Functional Foods." These bring enough nutrition per calorie that they are WORTH eating, while "Nonfunctional Foods" or "Dysfunctional foods" like this Mac and Cheese product bring tons of calories and so little USEFUL nutritional content that they are USELESS and indeed HARMFUL.

While it is true that some people have a genetic predisposition to be overweight, the fact of the matter is that the human body was never intended to live the way we do in the modern world: sitting at home, sitting in a car on the way to work and sitting at a desk at work. We evolved to toil and most people hardly move any more and that has dire consequences to our health – primarily our cardiovascular health. Add to that a poor diet consisting of foods high in trash calories and very low nutritional value laced with artificial cancer-causing chemicals and it is wonder that anyone makes it to the age of fifty any more.

If the problem begins with inactivity and poor diet, then correcting the diet is a good place to start. The primary focus is obviously to eat as many natural whole foods as possible rather than packaged and processed foods loaded with trash calories and laced with chemicals most of which have already been shown in numerous studies to be CANCER-CAUSING POISONS..

The problem with the natural whole foods diet is that many items actually have a lot of calories, most heavy plant foods like Sesame Seed Butter (a.k.a. Tahini,) Avocado, and Chocolate (100% Pure Cacao) are loaded with polyunsaturated fats. These are the "good kind" and they are also loaded with fat-soluble phytonutrients of enormous health benefit like the Omega-6 fatty acids. And some contain alpha-Linoleic Acid which is the only Omega-3 fatty acid found in plants (in reasonable amounts.)

Since seeds and nuts are the primary culprits of bringing large amounts of polyunsaturated fats and therefore calories, it would seem that in order to "go on a diet" a person would have to refrain from those foods until they have reached their target weight.

And if that is true, then there are many essential nutrients found primarily in the seeds and nuts that would be missing or in very low amounts in the other foods and that would mean that the dieter would have to get them from supplements instead of their natural sources.

Also there are several members of the "Big 43" essential nutrients that are very difficult to get from an all natural whole foods diet even if it is under no caloric limitations. Niacin, Choline, Riboflavin, Magnesium, Iron, Potassium, Zinc, Chromium and Calcium are particularly problematic. If a person has lactose intolerance or is trying to lose weight and is refraining from high saturated fat and cholesterol laden foods, Calcium may be impossible to get other than with a dietary supplement.

The goal is to lose weight and achieve OPTIMUM THRIVE-LEVEL health, so it is necessary to reduce caloric intake as much as is practical while at the same time maintaining the consumption of a satisfactory amount of food. One of the main problems with all diets is that while they feature reduced calories they also force the person to consume reduced portions which results in a "starvation diet" which can be miserable and frustrating. At the same time, unless those small portions are Enriched or Fortified (always with synthetic nutrients by the way,) there is no way they could bring all of the "Big 43" in at least 100% RDA amounts. And a person cannot possibly achieve OPTIMUM THRIVE-LEVEL health if they are not getting those essential nutrients in their proper amounts on a daily basis.

In the end, the human body is a machine, the most complex machine we know of, and it needs to absorb matter from the environment in order to function – to survive. We need in order of priority: Oxygen, Water, Calories, Protein (the Nine Essential Amino Acids, part of the Big 43,) and then the rest of the "Big 43" essential nutrients (Vitamins, Minerals and few others) and finally, the micronutrients (nutrients needed in very tiny amounts) and the phytonutrients (other organic molecules that the plants make for their own needs like Lycopene, which are very good for our health too) found in plants. If a person gets plenty of the first four but falls short of the rest of the Big 43 essential nutrients, they could survive for months maybe even years, but their health will decline gradually and they will get sick and eventually die. Even getting all of them in their proper amounts is not perfect because we still do not know how much Boron the body needs (a trace micronutrient) but we do know that plants must get it in trace amounts in order to grow and without it they stop growing and will eventually get sick and die. Since we are the descendants of Hunter-Gatherers that survived primarily on edible raw plant foods for millions of years, it stands to reason that we need trace amounts of Boron as well.

The bottom line here is to pursue a varied diet, low in calories, and to make certain that to get those Big 43 essential nutrients and also get a variety of plant foods that can provide the trace micronutrients and the wide variety of phytonutrients in them which science is currently studying and discovering that many of them are necessary as well. Since a reduced calorie diet will not cover all of the Big 43, then taking supplements will be a requirement until you reach your target weight and possibly beyond.

But the process of losing weight is distinct from maintaining ideal weight. So eventually you can go back to eating other heavier foods that are loaded with nutrients once you reach your target weight and learn how to eat a proper diet (which this book is all about.)

It is important to realize that being thin is not equal to being healthy. People with anorexia are thin, but far from healthy mainly because being thin becomes an obsession and they are only concerned with that; not with being healthy. So it is likely that very few of them ever take the time to learn about the Big 43 or make sure they are getting them in sufficient quantities and that is exactly why anorexia kills. It is also quite unnecessary to cut down to 3% body fat like athletes and body builders, but losing enough so that you FEEL better and ARE healthier, is the primary goal.

THE NATURAL WHOLE FOODS DIET
FOR LOSING WEIGHT

1) THE "NET NEGATIVE CALORIE" FOODS – All of these foods have very low calories: less than 30 cal/oz. If every food you eat all day contained 25 cal/oz, then you would have to eat 80 oz total to get 2,000 calories for the day – that's five pounds of food which very few people could eat. Cucumbers (skinned, because the skin is potentially bad for you) contain about 3.3 cal/oz. and it would take 36 pounds of them to get 2,000 calories and no one can eat that much in a day.

2) FRESH FRUITS and VEGETABLES – Most fruits happen to be far lower in calories than you might expect and unless you suffer from diabetes, the fruits are good because they contain no fat (in general, there are exceptions) and never any cholesterol, and they provide antioxidants and essential nutrients, and each fruit has a unique array of phytochemicals, many of which have been shown in scientific studies to provide a wide range of measurable health benefits. Some of these will be featured in the lists in the upcoming chapters because they actually promote weight loss too.

3) THE "BIG 43" – Since a low calorie diet cannot include the seeds and nuts which bring Vitamin E, the Omega-3 Fatty Acid alpha-Linoleic Acid, and minerals like Selenium, Manganese, Zinc and Copper, taking supplements to make sure you get them all in their proper amounts daily will be necessary and these products are covered in a later chapter as well.

4) HOLISTIC FOODS AND HERBS – There are plenty of foods, spices and medicinal herbs that can and will facilitate weight loss through various functions: some enhance the metabolism, some stimulate the burning of stored fat, others prevent new calories from being stored as fat, while others improve circulation which in turn helps blood sugars reach more cells and get burned rather than piling up and getting stored as fat. Upcoming chapters will list all of these foods, spices and medicinal herbs that will promote weight loss and some of them are essential to the success of your weight loss effort.

CHAPTER 4 – NET NEGATIVE CALORIE FOODS

Aside from exercise, diet is the primary concern, specifically to reduce caloric intake, but at the same time avoiding smaller portions to the point of absurdity. It makes no sense to reduce caloric intake by reducing portion size until the person is constantly suffering from hunger. This not only makes any diet miserable, it makes it unsustainable and eventually the person will give in to those cravings for "real" food and go back to their old eating habits and the diet fails. In fact, this is one of the main reasons why all diets fail in the end.

The best approach is to avoid "going on a diet" entirely. Instead concentrate on CHANGING your diet away from the old one: high in trash calories, saturated fats, cholesterol, artificial chemical additives, and low in nutritional value; toward a new and superior one: low in trash calories, saturated fats, cholesterol, chemical additives, and high in nutritional value. And the most important change of all: a new dietary regimen that DOES NOT LIMIT your portion sizes in each meal and allows healthy snacking any time you feel the need.

There is little doubt that eating lots of very low calorie foods can still leave you unsatisfied, or you will get the urge to snack more often because your body has become accustomed to the average amount of calories you have been eating for years. The good news is that there are ways to deal with this issue that are quite effective.

Before we get into those specific remedies, this chapter will concentrate on the actual diet itself. More to the point, I will list many Net Negative Calorie foods and the calories they actually bring based on serving size. It is impractical to list the calories per ounce in foods because no one is going to set up a scale in their kitchen and weigh the portions of every food they eat. But there is trouble when listing the amount of calories per cup of a specific food because what exactly constitutes one cup of raw spinach? Should you mash the leaves down tightly, or just stack them loosely?

The important thing to remember about the majority of the Net Negative calorie foods is that they are, for the most part, so low in calories that the portion size doesn't matter very much because you could never eat enough to pose a problem.

THE NET NEGATIVE CALORIE FOODS

FOOD	Cal/oz	1 CUP, Cal.
1. Shirataki Noodles, Cooked	<1	160g, a few
2. Watercress, Raw, Chopped	3.0	34g, 3.7cal
3. Waxgourd, Boiled, Diced	3.0	175g, 19 cal
4. Bamboo Shoots, Cooked	3.1	120g, 13.3cal
5. Pickles, Chopped	3.1	143g, 15.7cal
6. Taro Shoots, Raw, Sliced	3.1	86g, 9.4cal
7. Napa Cabbage, Cooked	3.3	109g, 13.1cal

Net Negative Calories Foods List (cont.)

FOOD	Cal/oz	1 CUP
8. Bok Choy, Cooked	3.3	170g, 20.4cal
9. Cucumber, Peeled, Raw, Chopped	3.3	133g, 16.0 cal
10. New Zealand Spinach, Boiled	3.3	180g, 21.6 cal
11. Calabash Gourd, Cooked	3.6	146g, 19.0 cal
12. Summer Squash, avg. all kinds	3.6	210g, 27.3 cal
13. Lettuce, Iceberg, Raw, Shredded	3.9	72g, 10.1 cal
14. Radish, White, Raw, Chopped	3.9	100g, 14.0 cal
15. Escarole, Boiled	4.1	150g, 22 cal
16. Mustard Greens, Cooked	4.2	140g, 21.0 cal
17. Nopales, Cooked, Chopped	4.2	149g, 22.3 cal
18. Celery, Raw, Chopped	4.5	101g, 16.2 cal
19. Purslane, Raw	4.5	43g, 6.9 cal
20. Radish, Red, Raw, Chopped	4.5	116g, 18.6 cal
21. Yellow Squash, Raw	4.5	113g, 18 cal
22. Zucchini, Boiled, Chopped	4.5	180g, 28.8 cal
23. Green Beans, Cooked	4.7	NA
24. Endive, Raw, Chopped	4.8	50g, 8.6 cal
25. Celtuce, Raw	5.0	NA
26. Tomato, Red, Raw, Chopped	5.0	180g, 32.4 cal
Tomato, Red, Cooked, Diced	5.0	240g, 43.2 cal
Purslane, Boiled	5.1	115g, 21 cal
27. Asparagus, Cooked, Chopped	5.3	242g, 46.0 cal
28. Swiss Chard, Raw, Chopped	5.3	36g, 6.8 cal
29. Chayote, Raw, Chopped	5.3	132g, 25.1 cal
30. Turnip Greens, Cooked	5.3	144g, 27.4 cal
31. Malabar (Vine) Spinach, Raw	5.3	NA
32. Bitter Gourd, Cooked	5.4	124g, 24 cal
33. Bell Peppers, Raw, Chopped	5.6	149g, 29.8 cal
34. Pumpkin, Boiled, Mashed	5.6	245g, 49.0 cal
35. Amaranth Leaf, Cooked	5.8	132g, 27.7 cal
36. Mushrooms, Button, Raw	6.1	70g, 15.4 cal
37. Okra, Boiled, Chopped	6.1	80g, 17.6 cal
38. Dock, (Sorrel) Raw, Chopped	6.1	133g, 29 cal
39. Turnips, Boiled, Diced	6.1	156g, 34.3 cal
40. Cardoon, Boiled	6.2	NA
41. Beet Greens, Raw, Chopped	6.2	38g, 8.4 cal
42. Sauerkraut (Low sodium)	6.2	142g, 31.2 cal
43. Cabbage, Boiled, Shredded	6.4	150g, 34.6 cal
44. Cauliflower, Boiled, Chopped	6.4	62g, 14.3 cal
45. Radicchio, Raw, Shredded	6.4	40g, 9.2 cal
46. Spinach, Cooked, Chopped	6.4	180g, 41.4 cal
Spinach, Raw, Chopped	6.4	30g, 6.9 cal
47. Pimento, Canned	6.4	192g, 44 cal
48. Capers, Canned, 1 Tbsp	6.5	8.6g, 2 cal
Chayote, Boiled, Chopped	6.7	160g, 38.4 cal
49. Tomato Sauce (no salt)	6.7	245, 58.8 cal
50. Alfalfa Sprouts, Raw	6.8	33g, 8 cal

Net Negative Calories Foods List (cont.)

FOOD	Cal/oz	1 CUP
51. Arugula, Raw	7.0	20g, 5 cal
52. Borage, Boiled, Chopped	7.0	NA
Cabbage, Raw, Chopped	7.0	89g, 22.2 cal
Cauliflower, Raw, Chopped	7.0	100g, 25 cal
53. Mushroom, Jews Ear, Raw	7.0	99g, 24.7 cal
54. Rose Apple (Malay Apple)	7.0	NA
55. Collard Greens, Boiled	7.2	190g, 49.4 cal
56. Mushroom, Portabella, Raw	7.3	86g, 22.4 cal
57. Spirulina, Raw	7.3	NA
Mustard Greens, Raw, Chopped	7.5	56g, 15 cal
58. Celeriac, Boiled	7.6	155g, 41.9 cal
59. Egg Drop Soup (Restaurant)	7.6	241g, 65 cal
60. Kale, Boiled	7.8	130g, 36 cal
61. Hearts of Palm, Canned	7.8	146g, 41 cal
62. Broccoli, Raw	7.9	71g, 20 cal
63. Kohlrabi, Boiled, Diced	8.1	165g, 48 cal
64. Lime. (or Lemon) 1 avg. fruit	8.4	67g, 20 cal
65. Agar, Raw	8.4	80g, 24 cal
66. Jalapeño. Raw, Sliced	8.4	90g, 27.0 cal
67. Watermelon, Diced	8.4	154g, 46 cal
68. Rutabaga, Boiled, Cubes	8.4	170g, 51 cal
69. Grapefruit, Sections	8.4	230g, 69 cal
70. Bean Sprouts, Raw	8.5	104g, 31 cal
71. Chives, Raw	8.5	NA
72. Fennel (Bulb) Raw, Sliced	8.7	87g, 27 cal
73. Leeks, Boiled, Diced	8.7	104g, 32.4 cal
74. Snap beans, Green, Raw	8.7	NA
75. Star fruit, Raw, Diced	8.7	132g, 41 cal
76. Beets, Canned	8.7	170g, 53 cal
77. Acerola Berry, Raw	8.8	98g, 31 cal
78. Tomatillo, Raw, Chopped	8.9	132g, 42 cal
79. Onions, Raw, Chopped	8.9	148g, 47 cal
80. Strawberries, Raw, Sliced	8.9	166g, 53 cal
81. Wonton Soup (Restaurant)	8.9	223g, 71 cal
82. Cress, Raw	9.0	50g, 16 cal
83. Surinam Cherries	9.2	173g, 57 cal
84. Dandelion Greens, Boiled	9.3	105g, 35 cal
85. Cantaloupe, Raw, Diced	9.5	156g, 53 cal
86. Acorn Squash, Boiled, Mashed	9.5	245g, 83 cal
87. Fiddlehead Fern, Raw	9.5	NA
88. Carrots, Cooked, Sliced	9.7	156g, 54 cal
89. Eggplant, Boiled. Diced	9.9	99g, 35 cal
Broccoli, Boiled, Chopped	9.9	156g, 55 cal
90. Brussels Sprouts, Boiled	10.1	156g, 56 cal
91. Honeydew Melon, Raw	10.1	177g, 64 cal
92. Mandarins, Canned in juice	10.3	249g, 92 cal
93. Mori-Nu, Tofu, Silken, Lite Firm	10.4	NA

Net Negative Calories Foods List (cont.)

FOOD	Cal/oz	1 CUP
94. Jicama (Root) Cooked	10.6	100g, 38 cal
95. Pomelo, Raw	10.6	190g, 72.2 cal
96. Peaches, Raw, Sliced	10.9	154g, 60 cal
Carrots, Raw, Chopped	11.4	128g, 52 cal
97. Prickly Pear, Peeled, 1 Pad	11.8	19g, 8 cal
98. Kelp, Raw	11.9	80g, 34 cal
99. Lambsquarters Greens, Raw	12.0	NA
100. Blackberries, Raw	12.1	144g, 62 cal
101. Papaya, Raw, Chunks	12.1	145g, 62 cal
Onions, Boiled	12.3	210g, 92 cal
102. Cranberries, Raw	12.9	110g, 50.6 cal
103. Plums, Raw	12.9	165g, 76 cal
104. Yardlong Bean, Raw	13.2	91g, 43 cal
105. Orange, Raw, 1 med. fruit	13.3	131g, 62 cal
106. Apricot, Raw, Sliced	13.4	165g, 79 cal
107. Loquat, Raw, 1 med. fruit	14.0	16g, 8 cal
Kale, Raw, Chopped	14.0	67g, 33.5 cal
108. Pineapple, Raw, Chunks	14.1	165g, 83 cal
109. Mamey, Raw	14.3	NA
110. Egg, Whites, Raw*	14.5	243g, 126 cal
111. Raspberries, Raw	14.6	123g, 64 cal
112. Apples, Raw, Chopped	14.6	125g, 65 cal
113. Cape Gooseberries, Raw	14.8	140g, 74 cal
114. Artichoke, Boiled	14.9	168g, 89 cal
115. Luffa Gourd, Boiled	15.1	178g, 96 cal
116. Pollock, Raw, Fillet	15.6	77g. 43 cal
117. Chestnuts, Cooked	15.7	NA
118. Currants, Red, Raw	15.7	112g, 63 cal
119. Blueberries, Raw	15.9	148g, 84 cal
120. Quince, Raw	16.0	NA
121. Yogurt, Nonfat	16.5	NA
122. Drumstick Tree Leaves, Boiled	16.7	42g, 25 cal
123. Longan, Raw	16.8	NA
124. Jambolan, Raw	16.8	135g, 81 cal
125. Mango, Raw, Chunks	16.8	165g, 99 cal
126. Kiwi, Raw, Sliced	17.1	177g, 108 cal
127. Natal Plum, Raw	17.4	150g, 93 cal
128. Cherries, Raw, Pitted	17.6	154g, 97 cal
129. Lychees, Raw	18.4	190g, 125 cal
130. Soursop, Raw, Pulp	18.4	225g, 148 cal
131. Grapes, Raw (avg. all varieties)	18.8	92g, 61 cal
132. Guava, Raw, Diced	19.0	165g, 112 cal
133. Scallops, Raw	19.3	NA
134. Cod, Raw, Fillet	19.3	116g, 80 cal
135. Green Peas, Canned	19.4	170g, 118 cal
136. Oysters, Wild, Eastern, Canned	19.6	162g, 112 cal

* Raw egg whites are antinutritional. The data is for the raw separated egg white but they should be cooked.

Net Negative Calories Foods List (cont.)

FOOD	Cal/oz	1 CUP
137. Flounder, Raw, Fillet	19.6	163g, 114 cal
138. Parsnip, Boiled, Sliced	19.7	78g, 55 cal
139. Persimmon, Raw, 1 avg. fruit	19.7	168g, 118 cal
140. Fava beans, Canned	19.9	256g, 182 cal
141. Hominy, Canned	20.2	165g, 119 cal
142. Shallots, Raw	20.2	NA
143. Burdock Root, Raw, Chopped	20.2	118g, 85 cal
144. Cottage Cheese (1% Milk)	20.2	226g, 163 cal
145. Fig, Raw, 1 medium sized fruit	20.7	50g, 37 cal
146. Haddock, Raw, Fillet	20.7	193g, 143 cal
147. Lobster, Raw (Northern)	21.6	NA
148. Blackeye Peas, Canned	21.6	240g, 185 cal
149. Lima Beans, Canned	22.0	241g, 190 cal
150. Perch, Raw, Fillet	22.3	64g, 51 cal
151. Olives, Ripe, Canned	22.7	170g, 138 cal
152. Bulgur, Cooked	23.2	182g, 151 cal
153. Sapodilla, Raw, Pulp	23.2	241g, 200 cal
154. Alaska King Crab, 1 lg leg	23.4	172g, 144 cal
155. Mahi-mahi, Raw, Fillet	23.7	204g, 173 cal
156. Blue Crab, 1 avg. sized whole	24.0	21g, 16 cal
157. Dungeness Crab, 1 avg. whole	24.0	163g, 140 cal
Cod, Baked, Fillet	24.0	90g, 77 cal
158. Bananas, Raw, Mashed	24.9	225g, 200 cal
159. Sunfish, Raw, Fillet	25.0	48g, 43 cal
160. Whiting, Raw, Fillet	25.3	92g, 83 cal
161. Turtle (Black) Beans, Canned	25.4	240g, 218 cal
162. Sweet Potato, Baked w/Skin	25.5	200g, 180 cal
163. Halibut, Raw, Fillet	25.5	204g, 186 cal
164. Grouper, Raw, Fillet	25.7	259g, 238 cal
165. Buckwheat Groats, Roasted	25.8	168g, 155 cal
166. Walleye, Raw, Fillet	26.1	159g, 148 cal
167. Veal, Shank, Raw, 4oz	26.3	113g, 106 cal
168. Jackfruit, Raw, Diced	26.7	165g, 157 cal
169. Tilapia, Raw, Fillet	26.8	116g, 111 cal
170. Striped Bass, Raw, Fillet	27.1	159g, 154 cal
171. Water Chestnuts (Chinese) Raw	27.2	124g, 120 cal
172. Soba Noodles, Cooked	28.2	114g, 113 cal
173. Teff Grain, Cooked	28.3	252g, 255 cal
174. Snapper, Raw, Fillet	28.3	218g, 218 cal
175. Wild Rice, Cooked	28.4	164g, 166 cal
176. Amaranth Grain, Cooked	28.6	246g, 251 cal
177. Sea Trout, Raw, Fillet	29.2	238g, 248 cal
178. Catfish, Wild, Raw, Fillet	29.4	143g, 150 cal
179. Mung Beans, Cooked	29.4	202g, 210 cal
180. Shrimp, Raw, Mixed Species	29.7	NA

SOME ADDITIONAL EXCELLENT FUNCTIONAL FOODS

FOOD	Cal/oz	1 CUP
1. Turkey Breast, (Baked, 4oz)	30.2	113g, 122 cal
2. Goat, Raw (100% Lean Cuts)	30.5	100g, 109 cal
3. Tuna (light canned, 5oz)	32.4	142g, 162 cal
4. Lentils (cooked)	32.8	198g, 230 cal
5. Beef Liver (raw, 3oz)	37.8	85g, 113 cal
6. Clams, Canned	39.7	160g, 227
7. Yeast Extract Spread (1oz)	44.0	NA
8. Cod Liver Oil (1 teaspoon)	44.0	NA
9. Chicken Breast (Baked, 4oz)	46.1	113g, 185 cal
10. Chickpeas (canned)	46.4	165g, 269 cal
11. Mussels (steamed, 4oz)	48.7	113g, 195 cal
12. Beef Sirloin (97% Lean)	50.0	113g, 200 cal
13. Atlantic Mackerel (4oz)	57.5	113g, 230 cal
14. Dried Plums (pitted)	68.5	172g, 418 cal
15. Spirulina (Dried, 1 cup, 4oz)	81.2	113g, 325 cal
16. Wheat Germ (½ cup)	100.0	70g, 250 cal
17. Oats (precooked ½ cup)	107.1	40g, 150 cal
18. Parmesan Cheese (3oz)	110.0	85g, 330 cal
19. Chia Seeds (1 Tablespoon)	137.0	≈ 38 cal
20. Brazil Nuts (2 kernels)	183.0	≈ 30 cal

(Source of both lists: http://nutritiondata.self.com)

The Net Negative Calorie Food list includes 180 different foods under 30 calories per ounce; some have a second entry to show average caloric content of raw versus cooked. The main cause of the variation is the change in water content from cooking. Most foods high in water content like raw plants and fish lose water while cooking. When the analysis is done on the same weight of cooked food, the caloric content is higher, but when you start with a specific weight of the raw food, it has a specific caloric content and that will not change much when it is cooked even though the total weight of the drained food may go down. Included in the list are leafy greens, vegetables, fruits, a few dairy items and many meats (all of them are Complete Protein that brings all nine essential amino acids) although the majority are seafood.

It is interesting to note that the breakpoint for a food bringing 100 calories per cup is about 17 calories per ounce. Obviously the density of the food is involved in this factor but of the first 124 foods in the list (all below 17 calories per ounce,) the only food over 100 calories per cup is raw egg whites which are too high in cholesterol and should be avoided during a diet anyway.

This simply means that those foods below 17 calories per ounce are so low in calories that it would literally take TWENTY CUPS (5 quarts) of them to total 2,000 calories for the day. I have a fairly good appetite and there is no way I could eat that much food, even if it was twenty different items from that list. This is the true power of the Net Negative Calorie foods, they will let you eat as much as you want and still won't take you over the daily limit in calories.

NET NEGATIVE CALORIE FOODS BY THE CUP

For those who want unlimited serving sizes (like me) so that they can combat their cravings to eat, not by sitting in misery, but by actually eating good foods that bring very few calories, these all bring less than 51 calories per cup: **Watercress**, Raw, (3.7cal per cup), **Arugula**, Raw (5.0), **Swiss Chard**, Raw, (6.8), **Purslane**, Raw (6.9), **Spinach**, Raw, (6.9), **Alfalfa Sprouts**, Raw (8.0), **Beet Greens**, Raw, (8.4), **Endive**, Raw, (8.6), **Radicchio**, Raw, (9.2), **Taro Shoots**, Raw, (9.4), **Lettuce**, Iceberg, Raw, (10.1), **Napa Cabbage**, Cooked (13.1), **Bamboo Shoots**, Cooked (13.3), **Radish**, White, Raw, (14.0), **Cauliflower**, Boiled, (14.3), **Button Mushrooms,** Raw, (15.4), **Pickles**, Chopped (15.7), **Cucumber**, Peeled, Raw, (16.0), **Cress**, Raw (16.0), **Celery**, Raw, (16.2), **Okra**, Boiled, (17.6), **Yellow Squash**, Raw (18.0), **Radish**, Red, Raw, (18.6), **Waxgourd**, Boiled, (19.0), **Calabash Gourd**, Cooked (19.0), **Broccoli**, Raw (20.0), **Bok Choy**, Cooked (20.4), **Mustard Greens**, Cooked, (21.0), **New Zealand Spinach**, Boiled (21.6), **Escarole**, Boiled (22.0), **Nopales**, Cooked, (22.3), **Portabella Mushrooms,** Raw, (22.4), **Bitter Gourd**, Cooked (24.0), **Agar**, Raw (24.0), **Jews Ear Mushrooms**, Raw, (24.7), **Drumstick Tree Leaves**, Boiled (25.0), **Jalapeño**. Raw, (27.0), **Fennel Bulb,** Raw (27.0), **Summer Squash**, Cooked, avg. all kinds (27.3), **Turnip Greens**, Cooked (27.4), **Amaranth Leaves**, Cooked (27.7), **Zucchini**, Boiled, (28.8), **Dock** (Sorrel) Raw (29.0), **Bell Peppers**, Green, Raw (29.8), **Bean Sprouts** (Mung bean) Raw (31.0), **Acerola Berry**, Raw (31.0), **Sauerkraut** (31.2), **Tomato**, Red, Raw (32.4), **Leeks** (Root & stalks) Boiled (32.4), **Kale**, Raw (33.5), **Kelp**, Raw (34.0), **Turnips**, Boiled (34.3), **Cabbage**, Boiled (34.6), **Dandelion Greens**, Boiled (35.0), **Eggplant**, Boiled (35.0), **Jicama** (Root) Cooked (38.0), **Chayote**, Boiled (38.4), **Green Beans**, Cooked (40.0), **Hearts of Palm**, Canned (41.0), **Star Fruit**, Raw (41.0), **Spinach**, Cooked (41.4), **Celeriac**, Boiled (41.9), **Tomatillo**, Raw (42.0), **Yardlong Bean**, Raw (43.0), **Pimento**, Canned (44.0), **Asparagus**, Cooked (46.0), **Watermelon**, Diced (46.0), **Onions**, Raw (47.0), **Kohlrabi**, Boiled (48.0), **Pumpkin**, Boiled, Mashed (49.0), **Collard Greens**, Boiled (49.4), **Cranberries**, Raw (50.6)

That's 72 foods that bring less than 51 calories per cup. If you ate one cup each of all 72 of them during the day that would come close to filling a five gallon bucket and total about 1,860 calories which is PERFECT for the day!

There are some caveats to these foods, however. Some of them are actually loaded with essential nutrients like Vitamin K. You can exceed the RDA amount of Vitamin K from natural whole foods (but never from supplements) but not by huge amounts and not day after day and some of these foods like Collard Greens do indeed bring huge amounts (1045%RDA/cup) – so much that it could cause a problem eating them on a daily basis. But there are many foods that will not bring excess dangerous nutrients.

The following are foods that do not bring too much of the dangerous essential nutrients that could cause trouble in excess: 1) **Napa Cabbage**, 2) **Cucumber**, 3) **Lettuce**, 4) **Celery**, 5) **Zucchini**, 5) **Yellow Squash**, 6) **Bok Choy**, 7) **New Zealand Spinach**, 8) **Tomato**, 9 **Chayote**, 10**Bell Peppers**, 11 **Turnips**, 2) **Bean Sprouts**, 13) **Cauliflower**, 14) **Arugula**, 15) **Cabbage,** 16) **Button Mushrooms**, 17) **Portabella Mushrooms,** 18) **Agar,** 19) **Watermelon**, 20) **Grapefruit**, 21) **Beets**, 22) **Onions**, 23) **Cantaloupe**, 24) **Strawberries**, 25) **Acorn Squash**, 26) **Carrots**, 27) **Honeydew melon**, 28) **Mandarin,** 29) **Tangerine**, 30) **Jews Ear Mushrooms**, 31) **Acerola Berry**, 32) **Eggplant**, 33) **Cranberries.** You should still stay under four cups per day per food in the list, but that is 33 low calorie foods in which you can overindulge; enough to be able to stave off cravings without piling on calories and without getting into trouble from excess nutrients.

BEVERAGES

Another important part of a low calorie diet is the beverages. While most folks may like diet sodas, they are terrible for human health. The Carbonic Acid and other acids bother the digestive tract and many of the artificial colors, flavors and sweeteners are proven CARCINOGENS. If you do not have Diabetes, then the fruit juices are better choices even though they bring some calories, but 100% pure fruit juices with no chemical additives have no cancer-causing garbage in them and they bring valuable phytonutrients that are not only good for your health but they are also proven preventatives and curatives of everything from cardiovascular disease, to high blood pressure, to urinary tract infections to even some forms of cancer.

BEVERAGE	Cal/oz	1 CUP, cal.
1. Water (Best Drink on Earth)	0	226g, 0 cal
2. Tea, Dark, Unsweetened	0	227g, 0 cal
3. Coffee, Black, Unsweetened	0	227g, 0 cal
4. Low Sodium Original V-8	5.6	250g, 45 cal
5. Acerola Juice	6.4	242g, 55.7 cal
6. Lemon/Lime Juice	7.0	244g, 61.0 cal
7. Blackberry Juice	10.6	250g, 95.0 cal
8. Grapefruit Juice	10.9	247g, 96.0 cal
9. Milk, Skim, 1%	11.7	250g, 105 cal
10. Tangerine Juice	12.0	247g, 106 cal
11. Orange Juice	12.6	248g, 112 cal
12. Apple Juice	12.9	248g, 114 cal
13. Cranberry Juice	13.1	237g, 111 cal
14. Pineapple Juice	14.8	250g, 132 cut
15. Pomegranate Juice	15.1	249g, 134 cal
16. Cherry Juice	16.5	269g, 159 cal

Low Calorie Beverages (cont.)

BEVERAGE	Cal/oz	1 CUP, cal.
17. Passion Fruit Juice	16.8	247g, 148 cal
18. Whole Milk, 3.25% fat	17.1	244g, 149 cal
19. Grape Juice, 100% Pure (avg.)	18.6	253g, 152 cal
20. Prune Juice	19.9	256g, 182 cal

(Source of this list: http://nutritiondata.self.com)

Obviously Skim Milk has lower calories and is a logical choice but whole milk is not totally evil either. Most 100% Natural Fruit Juices are low calorie, and bring zero fat and zero cholesterol. Juice your own and get in on all of the powerful phytonutrients they contain.

THE BOTTOM LINE

Replacing high calorie foods especially those that are nothing but starch, saturated fat, and cholesterol, laced with chemicals and having very little nutritional value with foods that are far lower in calories and much higher in nutritional value is the key to a successful diet. One of the more difficult foods to eliminate is baked goods made from bleached white wheat flour and this comes from over eighty years of acclimatization: baked goods are high in calories and have extremely little nutritional value.

Many of the Net Negative Calorie foods are Superfoods like the Swiss Chard, Collard Greens and Broccoli. Many others have scientifically confirmed medicinal properties including Pineapple, Tomato, and many others. The goal is to replace high calorie, low quality mainstays like potatoes, rice and corn with far superior low calorie, high quality (i.e. holistic and nutritional) foods.

Instead of potatoes, try side dishes like Cauliflower, Beets, Turnips, or even Yams which are admittedly high in calories but also have proven medicinal properties. Instead of the usual beans like Pinto, Kidney, or Navy beans try Lima beans, Green beans, Black beans, or the legumes including Green peas, Blackeye peas, and Lentils which are a little higher in caloric content, but again bring far superior nutrition, medicinal properties and have a much higher Dietary Fiber content and a much lower Crude Fiber content than the typical beans. It is this high Crude Fiber content of most beans that makes them bad foods – they irritate the digestive tract, while Dietary Fiber helps the digestive tract and clings to cholesterol preventing it from being absorbed during the digestive process.

Armed with 180 Net Negative Calorie foods you can always use them as substitutions for foods that are higher in calories and there are 72 choices that bring less than 51 calories per cup and they can really allow you to lower you caloric intake while not forcing you to reduce the portion sizes and that is one of the big keys to success: you do not have to stop eating altogether which can be miserable and frustrating. Instead all you really have to do is stop eating the WRONG foods, but you can certainly eat plenty of these excellent low calorie alternatives.

Nutrient density is the measure of how much of a given nutrient is in the food per ounce and more importantly per calorie. Finding foods with high nutrient density per calorie is key to a successful Natural Whole Foods Diet for losing weight, because you still need to get all members of the "Big 43" essential nutrients in OPTIMUM THRIVE-LEVEL amounts on a daily basis. The Net Negative Calorie foods are intended to SAVE calories and give you room to consume those foods that bring more calories but also bring the essential nutrients that the body must have.

NUTRIENT DENSITIES OF THE BIG 43

Each nutrient's top food sources will be shown including how much (percentage of the RDA amount) per calorie, percentage per gram, how many calories it takes to get 100% RDA amount, and how much is in a standard serving; 1 cup for the plant foods, 3 ounces for meats, 3oz for seeds and nuts, and 8 fluid ounces (1 cup) for the beverages, unless the amount is otherwise stated.

1. VITAMIN A (beta-Carotene = 3mg, Retinol = 1.5mg) – Many health professionals are advising people to get some of their daily Vitamin A as Retinol which only comes from animal sources.[1]

FOOD	%/cal	%/g	100%	Amt.
Carrots (raw)	8.152	3.343	12.3 cal	428%
Butternut Squash (boiled)	5.573	2.238	17.9 cal	457%
Sweet Potato (baked w/skin)	4.272	3.845	23.4 cal	769%
Beef Liver (raw)	2.503	3.380	40.0 cal	285%
Cod Liver Oil (1tsp)	2.216	22.5	45.1 cal	90%*

* Amount in one teaspoon.[38][47][48][159][160]

It is clear to see that raw carrots are indeed the best source of Vitamin A, not per cup, but per calorie and that makes a big difference. It only takes about 12.3 calories of carrots to deliver 100% of your Vitamin A for the day as beta-Carotene. That's a little less than ¼ cup of raw chopped carrots, since one cup brings about 428%DV.

Cod Liver Oil delivers 22.5% of the RDA of Vitamin A per gram, it is incredibly dense by weight, but Cod Liver Oil is also very high in calories. Fortunately, only a teaspoon (about 44 calories) will deliver about 90%RDA of Vitamin A. It also delivers 113%RDA of Vitamin D3 and 888mg Omega-3 Fatty Acids DHA and EPA. It is one of the most nutrient dense "foods" in this list.

2. VITAMIN B1 – THIAMINE (1.5mg) – It is alright to exceed the RDA amount of this vitamin daily, but try to stay below 250%. It is a water soluble vitamin and the body will get rid of any excess.[2]

FOOD	%/cal	%/g	100%	Amt.
Yeast Extract Spread (1oz)	4.095	6.464	24.4 cal	181%
Spirulina (dried 4oz)	0.548	1.590	182 cal	178%
Wheat Germ (2.5oz)	0.347	1.250	288 cal	87%
Pork (lean, top loin)	0.213	0.420	469 cal	36%
Pistachios	0.098	0.560	1019 cal	42%*

Clearly the Nutrient Density of Yeast Extract Spread sold as "Marmite" or "Vegemite" is far above any other natural whole food. One ounce brings over 100% RDA not just of Thiamine but also Vitamin B2 – Riboflavin and Vitamin B3 – Niacin and it is only 44 calories. This is really the ONLY WAY to get these three vitamins in excellent amounts without committing to a ton of calories EACH in order to get them.[43][56][58][161][162]

3. VITAMIN B2 – RIBOFLAVIN (1.7mg) – Like the rest of the B vitamins, it is OK to get more than the RDA amount per day but try to stay below 250%.[3]

FOOD	%/cal	%/g	100%	Amt.
Yeast Extract Spread (1oz)	5.341	8.290	18.7 cal	235%
Beef Liver (raw)	1.194	1.587	83.7 cal	135%
Button Mushrooms (raw)*	1.086	0.294	92.0 cal	25%
Chicken Liver (raw)	0.897	1.023	111.5 cal	87%
Spirulina (dried)*	0.745	2.134	134.3 cal	242%

* Button Mushrooms (common white") serving size = 1 cup (3oz,) Spirulina (dried) serving size = 1 cup (4oz) [48][58][161][163][165]

This is an excellent opportunity to point out that some foods have a very good nutrient density in terms of Percent per Calorie, but not in terms of Percent per Gram. Plain white Button Mushrooms will provide 100% of your Riboflavin in just 92 calories which would take FOUR cups of them to do it. There is nothing wrong with eating that much because they are low calorie, but it is impractical.

4. VITAMIN B3 – NIACIN (20mg) – Niacin has a much larger RDA amount than the other B vitamins and is difficult to get from natural whole foods other than Yeast Extract Spread. Try to get 100% RDA daily. It is not necessary to overindulge in this B Vitamin.[4]

FOOD	%/cal	%/g	Cals	Amt.
Yeast Extract Spread (1oz)	3.091	4.797	32.3	136%
Chicken (breast w/o skin)	0.516	0.564	193.7	48%
Tuna (canned in water, 5oz)	0.512	0.585	195.2	83%
Beef Sirloin (5oz)	0.262	0.458	381.5	65%
Salmon (raw 4oz)	0.257	0.388	388.6	44%

Some seeds and nuts bring Niacin, but they are so high in calories (and have such low nutrient densities per calorie) that they are not practical.[42][61][161][164][166]

5. VITAMIN B5 – PANTOTHENIC ACID (10mg) – Found in nearly all foods but in small amounts so getting 100% can be a challenge.

FOOD	%/cal	%/g	Cals	Amt.
Button Mushrooms (raw)*	0.565	0.152	176.9	13%
Beef Liver (raw 3oz)	0.530	0.705	188.3	60%
Chicken Liver (raw 3oz)	0.525	0.599	190.2	51%
Cauliflower (boiled)	0.448	0.104	223.0	13%
Salmon (raw 4oz)	0.216	0.326	462.2	37%

* Button (common white) Mushrooms serving size = 1 cup (3oz)

Plants have a low nutritional density per gram. It would take over SEVEN cups of either raw Button Mushrooms or boiled Cauliflower to get 100% Vitamin B5.[5][42][48][163][165][168]

TOP RECOMMENDED VITAMIN B5 SUPPLEMENT
===

MANUFACTURER: NOW FOODS
PRODUCT NAME: PANTOTHENIC ACID 500MG
WEBSITE: www.nowfoods.com
PRODUCT PAGE: www.nowfoods.com/supplements/
pantothenic-acid-500-mg-capsules

Pantothenic Acid is one of the more difficult B Vitamins to get in 100% RDA amounts from natural whole foods. Rather than take a potentially expensive natural extract source B complex, as long as you take care of B1, B2, B3 and most of the B9 with Yeast Extract Spread ("Vegemite"), and include some high B9 and B12 foods in your diet then you might only need B5, B6, and B7 supplements.

6. VITAMIN B6 – PYRIDOXINE (2mg) – This is another very difficult vitamin to get in 100% amounts from natural whole foods.

FOOD	%/cal	%/g	Cals	Amt.
New Zealand Spinach (raw)	1.125	0.158	88.9	9%
Bok Choy (raw)	0.800	0.094	125	16%
Bell Peppers (raw)	0.551	0.173	181.2	16%
Cauliflower (cooked)	0.414	0.096	241.7	12%
Beef Liver (raw 3oz)	0.398	0.529	251.1	45%
Chicken Liver (raw)	0.371	0.423	269.4	36%
Okra (raw)	0.354	0.110	281.8	11%
Broccoli (boiled)	0.327	0.115	305.5	18%
Tuna (canned in water 5oz)	0.308	0.353	324.0	50%

I have included a few extras for this vitamin because it is a hassle to get from natural whole foods. New Zealand Spinach has the highest density per calorie, but it would take ELEVEN CUPS to get 100% Vitamin B6.[6][48][49][61][129][165][168][170][171][172]

TOP RECOMMENDED VITAMIN B6 SUPPLEMENT
===

MANUFACTURER: NOW FOODS
PRODUCT NAME: VITAMIN B-6 50MG TABLETS
WEBSITE: www.nowfoods.com
PRODUCT PAGE: www.nowfoods.com/supplements/
Vitamin-b-6-50mg-tablets

Be aware that this product brings 25 TIMES the Recommended Daily Allowance. However, researchers are finding that some of the established RDA's fall way short of what we actually need on a daily basis. I have found no mention of this regarding Vitamin B6 but very few products offering only Pyridoxine will have less than this amount in them, so you will have to decide for yourself if you want to invest in a dedicated supplement, invest in a complete high quality B Vitamin Complex based on natural extract sources of the vitamins or pursue it in natural whole foods which is the best way to get it, but admittedly very difficult to do

7. VITAMIN B7 – BIOTIN (RDA = 300mcg, CDV = 30mcg) – I will use the CDV – Consensus Daily Value for this vitamin throughout this book rather than the RDA which was established long ago and cannot be achieved through natural whole foods.[7]

FOOD	%/cal	%/g	Cals	Amt.
Tomato (raw)	0.750	0.134	133.3	24%
Carrots (raw)	0.384	0.156	260.0	20%
Almonds (dry roasted, 3oz)	0.370	2.175	270.2	185%
Onions	0.293	0.128	340.7	27%

One ounce of Almonds has 62%CDV and 166 calories. Carrots, Tomatoes and Onions can provide the rest.[31][38][130][173]

TOP RECOMMENDED VITAMIN B7 SUPPLEMENT
==

MANUFACTURER: NOW FOODS
PRODUCT NAME: BIOTIN 1000MCG CAPSULES
WEBSITE: www.nowfoods.com
PRODUCT PAGE: www.nowfoods.com/supplements/ biotin-1000-mcg-capsules

This is a huge dose of Biotin and it is a water-soluble vitamin that will likely be eliminated when it is introduced into the body in such excess. Also, taking it every few days may not have the desired effect: the body will dump it all on the day you take it and you will be back to having no Biotin in your body the next day. Therefore it might be worth it to shop around for a product with a lower quantity in it per pill. Many B complex supplements do not even include it, so check the product label and make sure it is in there.

8. VITAMIN B9 – FOLATE (400mcg) – Getting enough Folate each day is not hard if you pick the High Folate foods.[8]

FOOD	%/cal	%/g	Cals	Amt.
Spinach (raw)	2.142	0.500	46.6	15%
Asparagus (boiled)	1.675	0.374	59.7	67%
Yeast Extract Spread (1oz)	1.613	2.504	62.0	71%
Turnip Greens	1.448	0.291	69.0	42%
Chicken Liver (raw 3oz)	1.268	1.446	78.9	123%
Broccoli (cooked)	0.764	0.269	130.9	42%
Lentils (cooked)	0.391	0.450	255.5	90%

One cup of boiled Spinach brings 66% RDA of Folate. The very best source is Yeast Extract Spread because just 1 ounce brings greater than 100% RDA amounts of Vitamins B1, B2 and B3, plus a good start on your Folate for the day. Most High Folate foods, especially the beans and peas bring some calories, but they also bring other valuable essential nutrients including Dietary Fiber which has been shown to help lower cholesterol and reduce the risk of colon cancer.[49][64][66][161][165][169][174]

TOP RECOMMENDED VITAMIN B9 SUPPLEMENT
==

MANUFACTURER: NOW FOODS
PRODUCT NAME: METHYL FOLATE 1000MCG
WEBSITE: www.nowfoods.com
PRODUCT PAGE: www.nowfoods.com/supplements/ methyl-folate-1000-mcg-capsules

Recent studies have shown that a High Folate Diet reduces the risk of cancer, but taking Folate supplements does NOT have a measurable effect. That should be enough to encourage you to seek out foods high in Folate.

9. VITAMIN B12 – METHYLCOBALAMIN (6mcg) – Vitamin B12 is an "animal thing." It is needed by the brain and nerves of all animals, so plants don't make any. Synthetic Vitamin B12 is called Cyanocobalamin and it DOES NOT EXIST in nature. If you are going to take supplements they should be from natural extract sources ONLY. No 30 year studies have been done to determine the long term effects of any synthetic essential nutrient, so we don't know how safe any of them are; Cyanocobalamin does yield CYANIDE when the liver converts it so it should be avoided.[9]

FOOD	%/cal	%/g	Cals	Amt.
Clams (½ can, 3.25oz)	11.18	16.26	8.9	1498%
Beef Liver (raw 3oz)	7.345	9.758	13.6	830%
Oysters (canned 2oz)	4.736	3.174	21.1	180%
Chicken Liver (raw 3oz)	2.381	2.716	42.0	231%
Scallops (raw 4oz)	1.324	0.899	75.5	102%
Salmon (raw 4oz)	0.842	1.269	118.7	144%
Sardines (canned 4oz)	0.721	1.481	138.7	168%

Most experts agree that the RDA for Vitamin B12 is a bit low; you can get much more on a daily basis, but be careful of the other constituents in the foods. Clams are also very high in Iron – so high that eating large amounts of them daily could result in IRON TOXICITY which is devastating to the liver. Every other day for this amount would be safe. Since the only reliable natural whole food sources of Vitamin B12 are animal products, Vegans should definitely consider supplements that provide it as a form other than Cyanocobalamin and it may be difficult to find one not made from an animal source.[42][48][53][62][54][165][175]

TOP RECOMMENDED VITAMIN B12 SUPPLEMENT
==
MANUFACTURER: NOW FOODS
PRODUCT NAME: METHYL B-12 1000MCG LOZENGES
WEBSITE: www.nowfoods.com
PRODUCT PAGE: www.nowfoods.com/supplements/
Methyl-b-12-1000-mcg-lozenges

Don't be too alarmed about the amount of Vitamin B12 in each of these pills, studies are starting to show that we can use far more of the B vitamins on a daily basis than what the FDA recommends. This quality product from a reliable vendor provides it in the correct form: Methylcobalamin and according to the manufacturer it comes from a non-animal based source and it is suitable for Vegans.

VITAMIN B COMPLEX
For those who want to be sure that they are getting all of the B Vitamins the very best way to do that is with a high quality Vitamin B complex supplement. I never recommend multivitamins because they are not physically large enough to bring Vitamin A through

Zinc in their 100% RDA amounts, but a B Complex is highly recommended because it CAN bring all of them in at least 100% RDA amounts and chasing after all 8 of the B vitamins can be a hassle and cost a lot of calories from natural whole foods.

TOP RECOMMENDED VITAMIN B COMPLEX

==

MANUFACTURER: Garden of Life
PRODUCT NAME: VITAMIN CODE – RAW B COMPLEX
WEBSITE: www.gardenoflife.com
PRODUCT PAGE: www.gardenoflife.com/content/product/vitamin-code-raw-b-complex/

I doubt you will find a more complete (includes all 8 including Biotin, often left out of many B complex supplements, and all 8 are present in at least 100% RDA amounts) or higher quality (and all of them come from natural sources) product on the market.

10. VITAMIN C – L-ASCORBIC ACID (60mg) – Vitamin C is the most studied nutrient of all and the general consensus is that the RDA amount is DREADFULLY LOW for OPTIMUM THRIVE-LEVEL health. It is an antioxidant and it supports to eye, skin, cardiovascular and immune health.[11]

FOOD	%/cal	%/g	Cals	Amt.
Acerola Berry (raw)	87.37	27.96	1.14	2378%
Watercress (raw)	6.486	0.705	15.4	24%
Guava (raw)	5.607	3.806	17.8	628%
Bell Pepper (raw)	5.413	1.706	18.5	157%
Kale (raw, ½ cup)	4.000	2.000	25.0	68%
New Zealand Spinach (raw)	3.500	0.500	28.6	28%
Bok Choy (cooked)	2.950	0.347	33.9	59%
Cabbage (cooked)	2.685	0.627	37.2	94%
Kiwi (raw)	2.527	1.542	39.6	273%
Cauliflower (cooked)	2.517	0.584	39.7	73%
Broccoli (cooked)	2.450	0.865	40.7	135%

Acerola berries have the highest Vitamin C content of any natural food. Watercress is the second densest by percent per calorie, but it is mostly water, so a cup only brings 24% RDA amount. Guavas have a very high density in both %/cal and %/gram and are the densest readily available source of Vitamin C. All other foods including citrus have lower densities and didn't make the list. [35][37][49][67][97][118][129][168][170][171][176]

11. VITAMIN D3 – CHOLECALCIFEROL (10mcg) –

FOOD	%/cal	%/g	Cals	Amt.
Cod Liver Oil (1tsp)	2.825	28.25	35.4	113%
Salmon (raw, 4oz)	0.865	1.305	115.5	148%
Atlantic Mackerel (4oz)	0.434	0.881	230	100%
Sardines (canned 4oz)	0.326	0.670	306.5	76%
Milk (whole, 8oz)	0.164	0.098	608.3	24%

Vitamin D is an oil soluble vitamin and you should NOT EXCEED the RDA amount on a daily basis. Synthetics are of dubious quality in terms of bioavailability and safety. We might not need much –

the 10 micrograms is the second smallest RDA of the Big 43 – but
if you cannot get it from natural whole foods you should try to get
two 20 minute exposures of your face and arms to direct sunlight
without sunscreen; that will allow your skin to make enough and
you will be good for the day.[12][42][47][60][62][177]

12. VITAMIN E – TOCOPHEROLS & TOCOTRIENOLS (20mg) –

FOOD	%/cal	%/g	Cals	Amt.
Swiss Chard (raw)	0.628	0.125	159.1	22%
Bell Peppers (raw)	0.344	0.108	290.0	10%
Sunflower seed kernels	0.226	1.305	441.4	111%
Almonds	0.215	1.269	463.9	108%
Peanuts (or peanut butter)	0.078	0.458	1,269	39%

There are eight common forms of Vitamin E; most are found in
seeds and nuts which bring a lot of calories. Avoid synthetics (they
are possibly TOXIC, especially in excess) and do not overindulge
in foods high in this oil soluble vitamin; excesses have been linked
to possibly causing stroke. Two cups of Broccoli will bring around
30% RDA and 110 calories so getting your Vitamin E from plants
other than seeds and nuts is possible but could still be quite a
challenge and possibly end up bringing excessive amounts of
Vitamin K.[13][31][32][33][171][178]

TOP RECOMMENDED VITAMIN E SUPPLEMENTS
==
MANUFACTURER: JARROW FORMULAS
PRODUCT NAME: FAMIL-E
WEBSITE: www.jarrow.com
PRODUCT PAGE: www.jarrow.com/product/292/Famil-E
==
MANUFACTURER: NOW FOODS
PRODUCT NAME: VITAMIN E 200 IU MIXED
    TOCOPHEROLS SOFTGELS
WEBSITE: www.nowfoods.com
PRODUCT PAGE: www.nowfoods.com/supplements/vitamin-
    e-200-iu-mixed-tocopherols-softgels
==
MANUFACTURER: Dr. MERCOLA
PRODUCT NAME: MERCOLA VITAMIN E
WEBSITE: www.mercola.com
PRODUCT PAGE: https://products.mercola.com/vitamine/
These three products include many forms of Vitamin E and are
recommended for those trying to avoid seeds and nuts and the
excessive calories they bring. There is evidence that CHRONIC
EXCESS MAY CAUSE STROKE. Since 1 IU of Vitamin E is the
equivalent of about 0.667mg d-alpha-tocopherol or of 1 mg of dl-
alpha-tocopherol acetate, 200 IU = 133 mg or about 10 TIMES the
RDA amount. I would recommend only taking ONE softgel of the
Now Foods product PER WEEK to be on the safe side.

13. VITAMIN K1 – PHYLLOQUINONE (80mcg) – Most people avoid Vitamin K because they think it causes internal blood clots but it actually helps to PREVENT INTERNAL BLOOD CLOTS and it is also required for proper bone maintenance and shortages can lead to cardiovascular disease and osteoporosis.[14]

FOOD	%/cal	%/g	Cals	Amt.
Spinach (raw)	25.85	5.838	3.9	181%
Collard Greens (cooked)	21.32	5.500	4.7	1045%
Kale (raw)	20.41	10.20	4.9	347%
Swiss Chard (raw)	18.17	3.613	5.5	636%
Cabbage (boiled)	5.828	1.386	17.2	208%
Broccoli (boiled)	4.454	1.570	22.4	245%
Asparagus (cooked)	2.850	0.640	35.1	114%
Dried Plums	0.308	0.745	324.0	129%

Vitamin K is obviously a "plant thing" especially in the leaves. But the Dried Plums also bring plenty along with many other significant nutrients. This is another oil-soluble vitamin that should come from natural whole foods rather than supplements and it is far too easy to get from plants to mess with pills that could possibly be TOXIC. [37][49][66][67][174][178][179][180]

14. CALCIUM (1000mg) – Calcium is required by the nerves, brain, and blood vessels and they go through a lot of it on a daily basis. And the bones will release it back into the blood to fulfill the demands of these other systems, so if you are not getting enough in your diet this can definitely lead to bone loss and osteoporosis.

FOOD	%/cal	%/g	Cals	Amt.
Bok Choy (cooked)	0.800	0.094	125.0	16%
Collard Greens (cooked)	0.551	0.142	181.5	27%
Parmesan cheese (3oz)	0.303	1.175	330.0	100%
Swiss Chard (raw)	0.286	0.057	350.0	10%
Swiss Cheese (3oz)	0.207	0.776	481.8	66%
Yogurt (plain, 8fl.oz)	0.201	0.122	496.6	30%
Milk (whole)	0.188	0.115	532.1	28%

Vegans might be very interested in those three high density plants, but you should not exceed 2 cups per day of any combination of them because all three are loaded with Vitamin K and in extreme excesses that will cause trouble. One cup of boiled Cabbage brings about 7.5% Calcium and also about 200% Vitamin K. Two cups of Broccoli brings about 8% Calcium and also more than 200% Vitamin K. The bottom line here is that some plants can provide Calcium, but in doing so they will bring far too much Vitamin K; to the extent that it is impractical and dangerous. You can take mineral supplements like Calcium Citrate (one of the best) but no more than 500mg per pill twice a day and bear in mind that it blocks the absorption of Phosphorus, another essential mineral also in this list.[15][37][44][46][72][170][177][178][179]

15. CHLORINE (2500mg) – Chlorine is a requirement for the human body even though it is toxic to most other forms of life especially in high amounts and 2.5 grams per day is very high. It is used in some nerve communication, the creation of hydrochloric acid in the stomach and also normalizes osmotic pressures in all fluids throughout the body allowing the cells to absorb the nutrients they need and to expel waste molecules. Despite the medical industry's Anti-Sodium/Anti-Salt crusade we do still need 2500mg each of Sodium and Chlorine each day. If you no longer indulge in packaged and processed foods which have way too much poor quality salt (no Iodine) in them, you can go back to adding about HALF A TEASPOON of IODIZED or SEA SALT to your own foods (total for the day) and easily cover THREE members of the Big 43 (Sodium, Chlorine and Iodine) with zero calories.[16]

16. CHOLINE (550mg) – Choline is a confusing issue. About 50% of the population has a genetic predisposition for a higher methyl metabolism which in turn creates a much higher need for this essential nutrient. Many ailments including poor fat absorption in the digestive tract or liver disease can also lead to deficiency and Choline is related to the B vitamins and is needed by the brain and liver in particular.[10]

FOOD	%/cal	%/g	Cals	Amt.
Beef Liver (3oz)	0.442	0.588	226.0	50%
Scallops (raw, 4oz)	0.389	0.264	256.6	30%
Cauliflower (cooked)	0.379	0.088	263.6	11%
Swiss Chard (raw)	0.342	0.068	291.6	12%
Egg (hard boiled, 1.75oz)	0.324	0.500	308.0	25%
Chicken Liver (raw, 3oz)	0.309	0.352	323.3	30%
Broccoli (cooked)	0.273	0.096	366.6	15%
Brussels sprouts (cooked)	0.273	0.096	367.0	15%

No single food can bring the 100% RDA amount in a convenient serving size making Choline a real problem to get in sufficient amounts on a daily basis. You should make every effort to get at least half of it from natural whole foods and only take supplements to finish the job.[48][49][165][168][175][178][181][182]

TOP RECOMMENDED CHOLINE SUPPLEMENTS
==

MANUFACTURER: NOW FOODS
PRODUCT NAME: CHOLINE & INOSITOL, 500 MG, 100 CAPSULES
WEBSITE: www.nowfoods.com
PRODUCT PAGE: www.nowfoods.com/supplements/choline-inositol-500-mg-capsules
==

MANUFACTURER: NOW FOODS
PRODUCT NAME: ALPHA GPC, 300 MG, 60 CAPSULES
WEBSITE: www.nowfoods.com
PRODUCT PAGE: www.nowfoods.com/supplements/alpha-gpc-300-mg-veg-capsules

I recommend both products and you can alternate them taking one on Sunday, the next of Monday, etc, and although the Alpha-GPC is expensive from any vendor, it has been shown to pass across the blood-brain barrier and gives the brain cells this critical nutrient they need to create their neurotransmitters and is too important to ignore.

17. CHROMIUM (120mcg) – Although we only need this mineral in micrograms it is critical for regulating blood sugar and it plays an active role in insulin pathways. Without Chromium, our blood sugar regulatory and metabolism systems decline and can ultimately fail leading to Type II "Late onset" Diabetes which is extremely difficult to treat. Diabetes kills over 80,000 people in the U.S. every year and the numbers of new cases diagnosed each year is on the rise.

FOOD	%/cal	%/g	Cals	Amt.
Garlic (raw, 1 teaspoon)	1.200	2.400	83.3	12%
Broccoli (cooked)	0.963	0.339	103.7	53%
Romaine Lettuce (raw)	0.250	0.047	400.0	4%
Grape Juice (100% Pure)	0.210	0.130	475.0	32%
Green Beans (cooked)	0.136	0.044	733.3	6%
Tomato (raw)	0.125	0.022	800.0	4%
Oats (precooked, ½ cup)	0.098	0.375	1,013	15%

One cup of cooked broccoli, plus one cup of 100% Pure dark Grape Juice and one teaspoon of minced garlic per day will get you very close to the RDA of Chromium for the day, but drinking grape juice daily can have negative consequences on the kidneys. There is nothing wrong with the Broccoli and the garlic, but even though I love both I don't want to eat large amounts of them daily. This might be the one mineral that most people will need to get at least sometimes from a supplement.[17][49][50][68][99][173]

TOP RECOMMENDED CHROMIUM SUPPLEMENT
==
MANUFACTURER: JARROW FORMULAS
PRODUCT NAME: CHROMIUM GTF, 200 MCG, 100 CAPS
WEBSITE: www.jarrow.com
PRODUCT PAGE: www.jarrow.com/product/214/Chromium_ GTF

This product provides Chromium in fermented yeast rather than Chromium picolinate which is being questioned by the medical industry concerning its effectiveness and safety. The RDA is 120mcg (micrograms) which may be anywhere from 2 to 4 times what most studies and health professionals have determined that the average adult actually needs. As such, this product should be taken no more than once every other day although once every three to five days would be OK. That will help offset the expense.

18. COPPER (2mg) – Copper is in at least seven enzymes linked to energy metabolism and it is also involved in the construction of Collagen, the protein in hair and nails, but also used in the joints. Chronic deficiency can result in painful and swollen joints and ultimately arthritis. Once the damage is done it is very hard to reverse; it can take decades of proper nutrition. The irony is that a varied Natural Whole Foods Diet as laid out in "Getting the Big 43

The Natural Way – Vol.1" will bring plenty of Copper, while the average American diet is almost completely DEVOID of it.]18]

FOOD	%/cal	%/g	Cals	Amt.
Beef Liver (raw)	3.539	4.703	28.2	400%
Oysters (canned, 1oz)	3.263	2.186	30.6	62%
Spirulina (dried, 4oz)	1.052	3.015	95.0	342%
Chocolate (Baker's, 1oz)	0.321	1.587	311.1	45%
Sunflower Seed Kernels	0.159	0.917	628.2	78%

Copper like all minerals can become TOXIC in excess. Try to maintain an average daily intake of the 100% RDA amount. Many seeds and nuts bring some copper in a typical 3 ounce serving. Most people eating a varied natural whole food diet DO NOT NEED TO TAKE COPPER. You should check the foods you regularly consume for the amounts of Copper in them before considering a supplement.[32][48][53][57][58]

TOP RECOMMENDED COPPER SUPPLEMENT
===
MANUFACTURER: SOLGAR
PRODUCT NAME: CHELATED COPPER, 100 TABLETS
WEBSITE: www.solgar.com

19. IODINE (150mcg) – We only need this mineral in micrograms as well, but it is critical to Thyroid health and gets included in at least one hormone made by this gland which is then sent out into the blood stream for other cells in the body to receive as a signal for metabolic rate control; therefore ALL cells in the body actually depend on this rare mineral which WILL become TOXIC in excess which can be even MORE DANGEROUS than deficiency.[19] While there are a few Iodine-rich foods like Kelp, Scallops, Cod and Yogurt, the amounts in them can vary quite a lot especially in Kelp and the best way to get it is:
½ TEASPOON of IODIZED or SEA SALT

20. IRON (18mg) – Iron is difficult to get in 100% RDA amounts from natural whole foods. Beef Liver, generally considered "high" in Iron would take about 13 ounces to deliver 100% RDA amount which would also bring far too much Cholesterol. And while 100% Pure Dark Chocolate (Baker's unsweetened chocolate bars) are an excellent source, it brings way too many calories and Tannins (that's what makes it dark and bitter and Tannins are bad for your kidneys.)[20]

FOOD	%/cal	%/g	Cals	Amt.
Clams (canned)	0.970	1.410	103.0	120%
Swiss Chard (raw)	0.629	0.125	159.1	22%
Spirulina (dried 3oz)	0.541	1.552	184.8	132%
Bok Choy (cooked)	0.500	0.059	200.0	10%
Chicken Liver (raw)	0.433	0.494	231.0	42%
Beets (canned)	0.327	0.103	306.3	16%
Asparagus (steamed)	0.250	0.056	400.0	10%
Collard Greens (cooked)	0.245	0.063	408.3	12%
Pumpkin (canned)	0.229	0.078	436.8	19%

Nutrient Densities of Foods that Bring Iron (cont.)

FOOD	%/cal	%/g	Cals	Amt.
Mussels (raw)	0.221	0.379	453.5	43%
Beef Liver (raw)	0.212	0.282	470.8	24%
Dark Chocolate (4oz)	0.193	0.952	518.5	108%

After Clams the only convenient source of 100% of your daily amount of Iron is Spirulina. 5 cups of Swiss Chard will bring far too much Vitamin K and 3 ounces of Chicken Liver is already bringing 100% Daily Limit of Cholesterol. Bok Choy is an excellent low calorie food loaded with nutrients but TEN CUPS of anything is way too much.[48][54][57][58][165][170][174][178][179][183][184][185]

21. MAGNESIUM (400mg) – Magnesium is an electrolyte as well as a mineral involved in countless enzymes and other biological functions in cells throughout the body. We also happen to need a rather large amount of it on a daily basis which is what makes it so difficult to get from natural whole foods.[21]

FOOD	%/cal	%/g	Cals	Amt.
Swiss Chard (raw)	1.029	0.205	97.2	36%
Okra (raw)	0.452	0.145	221.4	14%
Yeast Extract Spread (1oz)	0.295	0.459	338.5	13%
Collard Greens (cooked)	0.204	0.053	490.0	10%
Pollock (raw, 4oz)	0.194	0.176	515.0	20%
Butternut Squash (cooked)	0.183	0.073	546.7	15%
Flax Seed (ground, ½ oz)	0.173	0.917	576.9	13%
Spirulina (3oz)	0.172	0.494	581.0	42%
Wheat Germ (2.4oz)	0.168	0.593	595.2	42%
Dark Chocolate (4oz)	0.164	0.811	608.7	92%
Pumpkin Seeds (4oz)	0.144	0.635	694.4	72%

A good source is Magnesium Citrate, sold in most stores as a liquid laxative. The dosage of these products is the entire 8 to 10 ounce bottle which will work as a strong laxative. However, these products all bring about 200mg of Magnesium per ounce. Add about 1 tablespoon to any tart fruit juice (it takes like limeade) on four different occasions during the course of the day and you will get about 2 oz of Magnesium Citrate that will bring about 400mg of Magnesium. Another good product is Milk of Magnesia. Since the active ingredient is Magnesium hydroxide, a strong base that neutralizes stomach acid, you should take one teaspoon twice a day spaced far away from meals and that will also deliver about 440mg of Magnesium. Do not mix either source of Magnesium together and do not mix them with other supplements.[43][55][57][58][144][159][161][172[[178][179][186]

22. MANGANESE (2mg) – Manganese is involved in countless enzymes and other metabolic processes in the body including the absorption of many other nutrients by the intestines. Manganese is a "plant thing" and ounce for ounce they need a lot more than we do which is why they can provide plenty of it.[22]

FOOD	%/cal	%/g	Cals	Amt.
New Zealand Spinach (raw)	2.250	0.317	44.4	18%

Nutrient Densities of Manganese (cont.)

FOOD	%/cal	%/g	Cals	Amt.
Mussels (steamed)	1.949	3.351	51.3	380%
Wheat Germ (precooked ½ cup)	1.872	6.603	53.4	468%
Okra (raw)	1.613	0.504	62.0	50%
Napa Cabbage (boiled)	0.846	0.102	118.2	11%
Collard Greens (cooked)	0.837	0.216	119.5	41%
Green Beans (canned)	0.813	0.097	123.1	13%
Pineapple (raw)	0.807	0.407	123.9	67%
Kale (raw)	0.765	0.382	130.8	13%
Swiss Chard (raw)	0.714	0.142	140.0	25%
Dark Chocolate (4oz)	0.414	2.046	241.4	232%
Spirulina (4oz)	0.326	0.935	306.6	106%
Chickpeas (canned)	0.312	0.511	320.2	84%
Sweet Potato (baked w/skin)	0.278	0.252	360.0	50%
Lentils (cooked)	0.213	0.247	469.4	49%

A tablespoon of Wheat Germ added to Oatmeal should put you on track to getting enough Manganese for the day.[43][57][58][63][64][67][129][160][172][178][179][185][187][188][189]

23. MOLYBDENUM (75mcg) – We only need this mineral in micrograms but, it is important and involved in our ability to utilize sulfur which is common in most foods. Low Molybdenum can lead to joint troubles and severe deficiency could be life-threatening.[23]

FOOD	%/cal	%/g	Cals	Amt.
Green Peas (canned)	1.627	1.129	61.5	192%
Lima Beans (canned)	1.579	1.245	63.3	300%
Lentils (boiled)	1.435	1.663	69.7	330%
Black Beans (canned)	1.261	1.141	79.3	275%
Chickpeas (canned)	1.004	1.642	99.6	270%
Cucumbers (raw)	0.750	0.090	133.3	12%
Tomato (raw)	0.625	0.112	160.0	20%
Oats (½ cup precooked)	0.427	1.612	234.4	64%
Bell Pepper (raw)	0.345	0.109	290.0	10%

Luckily the beans and peas are loaded with it; just 2 to 3 cups of them spaced throughout the week will easily cover Molybdenum. [63][64][68][70][128][171][173][190][191]

24. PHOSPHORUS (1000mg) – Phosphorus is found in many basic molecules found in all living cells on Earth and forms the cross-links of the base pairs in the DNA double helix. Because all organs are under a continuous renewal process of cells dying and being replaced, we need a large amount of Phosphorus on a daily basis. It is found in all foods, but usually not enough to satisfy our daily requirement.[24]

FOOD	%/cal	%/g	Cals	Amt.
Scallops (raw 4oz)	0.896	0.608	111.6	69%
Button Mushrooms (raw)	0.435	0.118	230.0	10%
Shrimp (raw 4oz)	0.370	0.441	270.0	50%
Broccoli (cooked)	0.273	0.096	366.7	15%
Asparagus (cooked)	0.250	0.056	400.0	10%
Chicken Liver (raw 3oz)	0.247	0.282	404.2	24%

Nutrient Densities of Phosphorus in Foods (cont.)

FOOD	%/cal	%/g	Cals	Amt.
Sardines (canned 4oz)	0.240	0.494	416.1	56%
Wheat Germ (2.5oz)	0.240	0.847	416.7	60%
Pollock (raw 4oz)	0.233	0.212	429.2	24%
Cod (raw 5oz)	0.217	0.176	460.0	25%
Brussels Spouts (cooked)	0.214	0.077	466.7	12%
Sunflower seeds	0.196	1.129	510.4	96%

All seeds and nuts have high densities in %/g but they do bring a lot of calories. I don't recommend a Phosphorus supplement other than Bone Meal which is Calcium Phosphate. If you plan to take this supplement be sure to get enough Chromium, Magnesium, Vitamin K and Lysine as well so that your body can properly utilize the Calcium. Those with weak kidneys are given a low Phosphorus diet, so before you increase your intake of this mineral, you should check your kidney health first.[32][43][49][62][163][165][174][175][182][186][192][193]

25. POTASSIUM (3500mg) – Potassium has the highest RDA amount of any Vitamin or Mineral at 3,500mg. It is essential for nerve communication, fluid/osmotic pressure in all tissues and lowers blood pressure.[25]

FOOD	%/cal	%/g	Cals	Amt.
Bok Choy (cooked)	0.650	0.076	153.8	13%
Swiss Chard (raw)	0.571	0.114	175.0	20%
Low Sodium Original V-8	0.511	0.101	195.7	23%
Button Mushrooms (raw)	0.478	0.129	209.1	11%
Yeast Extract Spread (1oz)	0.477	0.741	209.5	21%
Zucchini (cooked)	0.448	0.073	223.1	13%
Tomato (raw)	0.375	0.067	266.7	12%
Asparagus (cooked)	0.300	0.067	333.3	12%
Butternut Squash (boiled)	0.207	0.083	482.4	17%
Brussels Sprouts (cooked)	0.200	0.071	500.0	11%
Yams (boiled)	0.165	0.191	607.7	26%
Banana (raw 4.8oz)	0.116	0.103	864.3	14%

Most people are surprised to see that Bananas rank rather poorly against other foods and they actually come in #21 in my master list. However, they are widely available, inexpensive, most people like them, and they also bring plenty of Dietary Fiber and other essential nutrients and Catechins (powerful antioxidants that the brain cells happen to like.) Three 8 ounce cups of Campbell Soup Company brand Low Sodium Original V-8 and two large Bananas a day will bring you that huge 3,500mg of Potassium we need. But it can be harsh of the kidneys so ramp it up slowly over a period of about two weeks. Potassium supplements have a moratorium of 100mg per pill (that's just 2.8% RDA amount) and they are too DANGEROUS to take in larger quantities than that and can cause a HEART ATTACK. Although it is a hassle, stick to natural whole foods (and the V-8) to get your Potassium.[69][73][159][161][163][170][173][174][178][182][194][195]

26. SELENIUM (70mcg) – Selenium is prevalent in seafood which is one of the reasons why I believe we are all descendents of "fish-eaters" and not indiscriminate carnivores. This is another "weird" element that the Thyroid gland needs to make its hormones and any long term deficiency can severely compromise your health.[26]

FOOD	%/cal	%/g	Cals	Amt.
Brazil Nuts (1oz)	4.191	27.055	23.9	767%
Button Mushrooms (raw)	1.391	0.376	71.9	32%
Shrimp (raw 4oz)	0.756	0.899	132.4	102%
Mussels (steamed 4oz)	0.744	1.279	134.5	145%
Chicken Liver (raw)	0.680	0.776	147.0	66%
Cod (raw 5oz)	0.652	0.529	153.3	75%
Scallops (raw 4oz)	0.584	0.397	171.1	45%
Pollock (raw 4oz)	0.583	0.529	171.7	60%
Asparagus (cooked)	0.400	0.090	250.0	16%
Beef Liver (raw)	0.372	0.494	269.0	42%
Sardines (canned 4oz)	0.361	0.741	277.4	84%
Beef Sirloin (5oz)	0.323	0.564	310.0	80%
Wheat Germ (2.5oz)	0.320	1.129	312.5	80%
Atlantic Mackerel (raw 4oz)	0.313	0.635	319.4	72%
Pork (top loin 5oz)	0.308	0.600	324.7	85%
Turkey (light w/o skin 6oz)	0.295	0.459	338.5	78%

Brazil Nuts have the highest concentration of Selenium of any food; just two Brazil nut kernels bring about 100% RDA of this critical mineral and are the best way to get it from a natural whole food source.[43][48][60][62][65][162][163][165][166][174][175][185][183][192][193][196]

27. SODIUM (2500mg) – Sodium is a critical requirement for maintaining proper blood serum electrolyte balance as well as supporting nerve communication. Excesses are to be avoided as this can result in high blood pressure.[27] The easiest way to get it is to avoid all processed and packaged foods with added salt which has no iodine in it and then add:

½ TEASPOON OF IODIZED OR SEA SALT to your food daily

28. SULFUR (No RDA) – Although Sulfur has no RDA it is an essential nutrient and all foods have some sulfur in them. But many plants are significant sources not only of sulfur but also a large category of phytonutrients called the Glucosinolates which are sulfur-containing compounds that include antioxidants as well as many other compounds that have been shown to possess significant health promoting properties.[28]

GOOD SOURCES OF SULFUR: GARLIC, ONIONS, BROCCOLI, CABBAGE, BOK CHOY, CAULIFLOWER, BLACK PEPPER, MUSTARD, CHIVES, SHALLOTS, LEEKS, EGGS, FISH.

These are all easily recognized as the "stinky" foods, because they are high in sulfur and it is easy to get enough of this mineral each day. Many are loaded with other nutrients and Glucosinolates (sulfur compounds) that have a wide range of surprising health benefits.

29. ZINC (15mg) – We need almost as much Zinc as we do Iron, but it is not nearly as common in natural foods which makes it a real challenge to get enough each day.[29]

FOOD	%/cal	%/g	Cals	Amt.
Oysters (canned 1oz)	8.947	5.996	11.2	170%
Veal (raw 4oz)	0.258	0.273	387.1	31%
Asparagus (cooked)	0.250	0.056	400.0	10%
Wheat Germ (2.5oz)	0.240	0.847	416.7	60%
Beef Sirloin (5oz)	0.222	0.388	450.9	55%
Lamb (5oz)	0.221	0.529	453.3	75%
Scallops (raw 4oz)	0.208	0.141	481.3	16%
Beef Liver (raw)	0.186	0.247	538.1	21%
Chicken Liver (raw)	0.155	0.176	646.7	15%
Pumpkin Seeds	0.152	0.670	657.9	57%

No natural whole food even comes close to Oysters in terms of both % per calorie and % per gram of Zinc. Pumpkin seeds have the highest concentration of any readily available plant food and would still take over 650 calories to fulfill your daily requirement of this important mineral.[43][48][53][55][74][165][166][174]]175][197]

TOP RECOMMENDED ZINC SUPPLEMENTS
==

MANUFACTURER: NOW FOODS
PRODUCT NAME: L-OPTIZINC 30 MG
WEBSITE: www.nowfoods.com
PRODUCT PAGE: www.nowfoods.com/supplements/
l-optizinc-30-mg-veg-capsules
==

MANUFACTURER: GARDEN OF LIFE
PRODUCT NAME: VITAMIN CODE RAW ZINC
WEBSITE: www.gardenoflife.com
PRODUCT PAGE: www.gardenoflife.com/content/product/
vitamin-code-raw-zinc/

Both of these quality products provide Zinc in a highly available form. The Now Foods product is a synthetic chelate shown to be very well absorbed in the digestive tract and the Garden of Life product is a natural source extract of the highest quality.

30. ALPHA-LINOLEIC ACID (est. 500+ mg) – Numerous studies have demonstrated that the Omega-3 Fatty Acids like ALA are essential nutrients and act as anti-inflammatory agents that can reduce the risk of cardiovascular disease.[59]

FOOD	mg/cal	mg/g	Cals	Amt.
Chia Seed (1 Tbsp)	64.66	346.67	38	2457mg
Flax Seed (2 Tbsp)	42.53	225.04	75	3190mg
Walnuts (1oz)	14.56	93.97	183	2664mg

These are by far the three most concentrated sources of the plant Omega-3 Fatty Acid ALA. We can convert ALA into DHA and EPA (the next two essential nutrients in this list) but we still do not know if the body can produce enough daily to keep up with demand. It is an excellent idea to add alpha-Linoleic Acid to your daily diet. Most health professionals advise DHA and EPA as well.[30][144][145]

31. DOCOSAHEXAENOIC ACID (DHA, always found together with EPA, est. 520mg) – Like ALA, DHA and EPA are listed by the literal amounts in milligrams found in the foods rather than percentages of the RDA. It appears that the FDA is going to issue an RDA for these two essential nutrients at 520mg/day.

FOOD	mg/cal	mg/g	Cals	Amt.
Cod Liver Oil (1 tsp)	20.181	222.000	44	888
Atlantic Mackerel (4oz)	13.043	26.455	230	3000
Salmon (sockeye, 4oz)	7.392	11.146	171	1264
Sardines (canned, 4oz)	7.082	14.550	233	1650
Tuna (light canned 5oz)	2.469	2.822	162	400

DHA and EPA are obviously a "fish thing" and another factor in my conclusion that all modern humans are the descendents of "fish-eaters" rather than indiscriminate carnivores. No other foods on Earth, except seafood, bring DHA and EPA in the amounts we need in our diet. I have found one fern that has just a few mg of EPA in a typical serving size. In order to get enough from that plant source you would have to defoliate a ¼ acre/day. Evidence suggests that we should consume enough DHA and EPA so that the RATIO of Omega-6 Fatty Acids (found in seeds, nuts and vegetable oils in large amounts) to the Omega-3 Fatty Acids should be no higher than 5 to1 with 2 to 1 being ideal in order to reap the health benefits from both kinds of nutritional fatty acids. Because of this and the fact that most people consume a lot of the Omega-6 Fatty acids (some are prevalent even in some fruits like Pomegranate) and rarely eat the richest sea foods, I recommend taking a DHA/EPA OMEGA-3 FATTY ACID supplement on a daily basis.[42][59][60][61][62]

TOP RECOMMENDED OMEGA-3 SUPPLEMENTS
==

MANUFACTURER: Any Reputable Brand
PRODUCT NAME: COD LIVER OIL (1Tsp/day)
==

MANUFACTURER: Any Reputable Brand
PRODUCT NAME: DHA/EPA OMEGA-3 (520mg)

Cod Liver Oil is one of the best natural supplements you could take bringing Vitamin A as Retinol, Vitamin D3, and 888mg of the Omega-3 Fatty Acids DHA and EPA. Fish Oil pills are acceptable but some health professionals have noted that Krill oil pills may be contaminated. Bear in mind that Olive oil is the only salad dressing you should use (Oil and Vinegar) and it is loaded with Omega-6's which will need to be balanced by Omega-3's as well. The Omega-3's are considered very safe nutrients; overdosing, even extreme amounts, has shown no adverse reactions or toxic effects.[59][71]

32. EICOSAPENTAENOIC ACID (EPA, See DHA above)

33. ISOLEUCINE (19mg/kg) – This is the first of the nine essential amino acids that must be consumed in sufficient quantities on a daily basis because the body cannot manufacture it. This amino acid is involved in the formation of hemoglobin in the blood and muscle growth especially in children.[52]

34. HISTIDINE (14mg/kg) – Histidine is involved in detoxification of the body and is another critical component required to maintain healthy brain function.[52]

35. LEUCINE (42mg/kg) – Leucine, like all amino acids, is an integral part of many proteins used by all cells in the body but it is also used to moderate insulin levels and helps regulate blood sugar levels in the blood. [52]

36. LYSINE (38mg/kg) – Lysine is considered the "animal amino acid" and most plant proteins have very low amounts and we need a lot of it daily. Lysine is necessary for proper utilization of calcium in the body and promotes bone health.[52]

37. METHIONINE (+ Cysteine 19mg/kg total of both) – Methionine is a critical component of bone cartilage and helps in producing Creatine, a precursor to ADP – Adenosine Triphosphate – the main fuel used by muscle cells. The actual RDA is 19mg/kg of both Methionine and Cysteine which should both be acquired in proper amounts: about 13mg/kg of Methionine and 6mg/kg of Cysteine which alone is not considered essential (we can make it.) Methionine contains a sulfur atom and is generally deficient in plant proteins.[52]

38. PHENYLALANINE (+ Tyrosine 33mg/kg total of both) – Phenylalanine is used by the Thyroid to produce its hormones and a dietary lack can result in similar deficiency syndromes to either Iodine and/or Selenium. Tyrosine which in not essential (we can make it) is involved in the construction of the Thyroid hormones and possibly other uses of Phenylalanine as well. The ideal ratio of the two amino acids is roughly 1 to 1.[52]

39. THREONINE (20mg/kg) – Threonine is a critical component of the central nervous system and it is important for heart and liver health and also plays a key role in the immune system.[52]

40. TRYPTOPHAN (5mg/kg) – Tryptophan does NOT cause drowsiness. If that were true then Chicken, which has a higher concentration of this important amino acid than Turkey, would make everyone sleepy too. Since it doesn't, Tryptophan cannot be the culprit. Ironically, Tryptophan is an important nutrient for the brain and adequate supplies are needed for the brain to build its neurotransmitter chemicals and maintain alertness and sharp memory. Chronic deficiency will lead to cognitive decline, memory loss, mood changes, and sluggishness – the exact opposite of what most people believe. People get drowsy after Thanksgiving dinner because we generally eat far too much food especially the Turkey and massive overindulgence in protein and calories will make you drowsy.[52]

41. VALINE (24mg/kg) – Valine is well known to athletes and body builders and is necessary for muscle health and is involved in muscle growth, repair and endurance.[52]

COMPLETE PROTEIN (50g/day) – Getting all nine essential amino acids in sufficient amounts per day is a complex issue because the RDA's are based on body weight which is a "one size fits all" recommendation and no two protein sources provide them in the same ratios to each other. The following table uses the amounts of Complete Protein as a percentage of the RDA amount (50 grams) although this is still not reliable because of the ratios of the nine essential amino acids found in the specific food. And all foods calculations are done on one ounce and the amount of Protein is given in Grams rather than the RDA percentage.

FOOD	%/cal	%/g	Cals, oz	g/oz
*Tuna (light, canned)	0.437	0.501	228.9, 7.0	7.1g
*Cod (Atlantic)	0.435	0.353	230.0, 10	5.0g
Chicken Breast	0.422	0.459	236.9, 7.7	6.5g
*Pollock	0.419	0.381	238.9, 9.3	5.4g
*Venison	0.405	0.600	247.1, 5.9	8.5g
Spirulina (dried)	0.397	1.136	252.2, 3.1	16.1g
Shrimp	0.384	0.402	260.5, 8.8	5.7g
*Turkey Breast	0.382	0.593	261.9, 6.0	8.4g
Goat	0.380	0.409	262.9, 8.6	5.8g
Scallops	0.368	0.409	271.6, 8.6	5.4g
*Veal	0.358	0.381	279.6, 9.3	7.2g
Clams (canned)	0.348	0.508	287.5, 6.9	8.6g
Beef Sirloin	0.347	0.607	288.4, 5.8	5.7g
Beef Liver	0.302	0.402	331.6, 8.8	4.7g
*Chicken Liver	0.289	0.332	345, 10.6	6.1g
Salmon (sockeye)	0.285	0.430	350.8, 8.2	6.7g
Mussels	0.278	0.473	359.7, 7.5	7.4g
*Pork (top loin)	0.268	0.522	373.0, 6.8	6.9g
Sardines (canned)	0.237	0.487	421.7, 7.2	2.0g
Oysters (canned, boiled)	0.207	0.141	482.5, 25	4.6g
Ham (deli, avg. 11 fat)	0.202	0.325	495, 10.9	7.1g

* Forms of Complete Protein with the best ratios of the nine essential amino acids[42][48][53][54][58][61][62][162][164][165][166][175][185][186][192][193][196][197][198][199][200]

This table demonstrates just how good Tuna fish is for your health. Aside from its nutritional value, it is the densest source of protein per calorie of any readily available food and it has an excellent Complete Protein Essential Amino Acid profile (excellent ratios of all nine) and all nutrient content values in this book are based on the average amounts found in any quality brand of canned light Tuna in water. To get 100% RDA of Complete Protein would take just 228 calories or about 7oz which is admittedly a bit excessive for some folks. A good rule for the foods with ideal Complete Protein profiles (marked with an asterisk) is:

(Weight in pounds ÷ 200) x Amt. from 4th column = Amt. needed
Example: A Person Weighing 140lb for Tuna:
        (140lb ÷ 200) x 7.0oz = 4.9oz

Therefore, a 140lb person would get all of the nine essential amino acids they need for the day from one 5oz can of chunk light Tuna in water.

42. ANTIOXIDANTS (No RDA) – This is a huge category of phytochemicals. They are basically unique to plants although animals do make them and the human liver manufactures one for the body called Glutathione. Most folks are aware that Vitamin C is a powerful antioxidant, but beta-Carotene commonly found in many plants is 25 TIMES more potent. And Lycopene, which makes tomatoes and watermelon pulp red, is 40 TIMES more potent than Vitamin C. There has been a lot of hype about the antioxidants but it is well deserved. Antioxidants "relieve oxidative stress" in virtually all cells in the body which in turn makes every organ system healthier by reducing cell death and increasing the vitality of the cells which makes the organs healthier and brings them up to OPTIMUM THRIVE-LEVEL health and performance.

"Relieve oxidative stress" in all cells means that antioxidants neutralize the metabolic waste by-products caused by burning carbohydrates and proteins. Proteins in particular are very dirty burning fuels that produce very toxic waste in the cells compared to the carbs which also produce toxic waste by-products. These waste by-products can lead to a decline in the performance of the cell and even kill it when left unchecked. Unmanaged diets low in antioxidant-rich foods literally causes a build-up of toxic oxidants in all tissues and no magical detox product can fix this – only the antioxidants can transform your body from an oxidant-rich environment to a clean environment low in oxidants.

Numerous studies have shown that the antioxidants do serve as detoxification agents that improve the health and performance of literally every organ system in the body and reduce the risks of (help prevent) and can even ameliorate the effects of just about every one of the BIG SEVEN modern deadly epidemic plagues including but certainly not limited to: 1) Cardiovascular Disease, 2) High Blood Pressure, 3) High Cholesterol, 4) Alzheimer's disease, 5) Type II Diabetes, 6) Stroke, and 7) Cancer.

And the vast majority of all cases of these terrible afflictions are the result of chronic poor diet starting with a shortage of antioxidant-rich foods. These foods bring many other essential nutrients as well as their own specific phytonutrients that help stave off these diseases as well.

The worst of all modern plagues is Cancer which CREATES and THRIVES in OXIDANT-RICH environments. It is therefore no coincidence that oxidant-rich environments ENCOURAGE its formation, growth, proliferation and spread while antioxidant-rich environments can dramatically reduce the risk of its formation and slow its progress. Do yourself a favor and load up on antioxidants.

I have used the ORAC (Oxygen Radical Absorption Capacity) Scores of each food despite the fact that this is considered an obsolete form of measurement. This is basically because no two antioxidants are the same. Nevertheless, the same amount of each food is used in the measurement process (100 grams) and it provides a convenient method of comparing the foods side-by-side. There are other methods of measuring the antioxidants in foods now, but they are not really that much better.[34]

FOOD	ORAC	O/cal	O/g	Oz.	Cal
1. Cranberries	9090	196.08	90.90	3.5	46
2. Black Plums	7581	164.02	75.81	5.8	76
3. Strawberries	4302	132.57	43.02	5	46
4. Dark chocolate	49944	101.14	499.44	4	560
5. Artichokes (cooked)	4760	91.49	47.60	4	59
6. Red Delicious Apple	4275	82.04	42.75	4.4	65
7. Blueberries	4669	81.94	46.69	5.2	84
8. Arugula	1904	75.57	19.04	0.7	5
9. Asparagus (cooked)	1644	73.41	16.44	6.3	40
10. Black beans (can)	6416	70.92	64.16	8.5	218
11. Spinach	1513	67.40	15.13	1.1	7
12. Bean Sprouts	1510	64.21	15.10	1.2	8
13. Lentils	7282	62.83	72.82	7	230
14. Broccoli (cooked)	2160	61.24	21.60	5.5	55
15. Blackeye Peas	4343	56.57	43.43	8.5	185
16. Beets (canned)	1776	56.51	17.76	5.5	49
17. Swiss Chard	1108	55.64	11.08	6.2	35
18. Pomegranate	4479	53.79	44.79	6.1	144
19. Grapefruit (red)	1640	51.03	16.40	9	82
20. Figs	3383	45.36	33.83	3.5	74
21. Brussels sprouts*	1330	37.03	13.30	5.5	56
22. Cabbage (boiled)	856	36.75	8.56	5.3	35
23. Kale	1770	35.42	17.70	1.2	17
24. Dried Plums	8059	33.34	80.59	6.1	418
25. Celery	552	32.22	5.52	3.5	17
26. Cauliflower (cook)	739	31.79	7.39	4.4	29
27. Lettuce (Iceberg)	438	31.04	4.38	2.5	10
28. Tangerine	1627	30.90	16.27	6.9	103
29. Bell Peppers	935	29.71	9.35	3.25	29
30. Pecans	17940	25.56	179.40	3	597
31. Button Mushrooms	691	25.55	6.91	3	23
32. Grapes (black)	1746	25.23	17.46	5.3	104
33. Green beans (can)	290	24.41	2.90	4.75	16
34. Tomato (cooked)	423	23.61	4.23	6.3	32
35. Sweet Potato*	2115	23.32	21.15	7	180
36. Apricot	1110	22.68	11.10	4.9	68
37. Mango	1300	21.59	13.00	5.8	99
38. Walnuts (English)	13541	20.98	135.41	1	183
39. Guava	1422	20.88	14.22	5.8	112
40. Pineapple	943	18.68	9.43	5.8	83
41. Leeks	569	17.64	5.69	3.5	32
42. Carrots	697	17.10	6.97	4.5	52
43. Pumpkin (canned)	483	14.19	4.83	8.6	83
44. Kiwi	862	14.14	8.62	6.25	108

Antioxidant ORAC Densities (cont.)

FOOD	ORAC	O/cal	O/g	Oz.	Cal
45. Grapefruit (red)	1640	51.03	16.40	9	82
46. Onions (Sweet)	614	14.00	6.14	7.4	92
47. Pistachios	7675	13.60	76.75	3	480
48. Avocado	1922	12.03	19.22	5.3	240
49. Cucumber	140	11.66	1.40	4.7	16
50. Raisins (seedless)	3406	11.27	34.06	3.5	300

* Values are for steamed Brussels sprouts, baked Sweet Potato

These are the Top 50 foods with the highest ORAC density per calorie. These foods deliver the most antioxidant power while also delivering the fewest calories. All foods above are for the RAW food unless otherwise stated. Included is the weight of a 1 CUP serving (other than seeds and nuts) and the calories it contains. In order to get as much antioxidant power as any given food, every food listed below it would take more calories to do it. However, you might not want to consume 560 calories of Dark Chocolate, and many foods below it do bring far fewer calories while bringing excellent antioxidant power like Artichokes, Apples, Blueberries and Arugula.[34]

However, the highest antioxidant density of all foods belongs to the dried spices. They have far higher antioxidant densities per calorie than any of the conventional foods and you should use them liberally in your cooking to take advantage of their incredibly high antioxidant potency and their powerful and often unique phytonutrients that deliver a wide range of proven health benefits.

THE SPICE RACK – THE ANTIOXIDANT POWERHOUSE
Basil (ORAC Score: 61,063 dried, 4,805 fresh), **Black Pepper** (34,053 ground), **Cayenne Pepper** (19,671 ground), **Chili Powder** (23,636), **Cilantro** (5,141 fresh), **Cinnamon** (131,420 ground), **Cloves** (290,283 ground), **Cumin** (50,372), **Curry Powder** (48,504), **Dill Weed** (4,392 fresh), **Garlic** (6,665 dried; 5,708 fresh), **Ginger** (39,041 ground, 14,840 raw), **Lemon Balm** (5,997 fresh), **Marjoram** (92,310 dried), **Nutmeg** (69,640 ground), **Oregano** (13,970 fresh; 175,295 dried), **Paprika** (21,932), **Parsley** (73,670 dried), **Peppermint Leaves** (160,820 dried, 13,978 fresh), **Rosemary** (165,280 dried; 11,070 fresh), **Saffron** (whole, 20,580), **Sage** (119,929 dried; 32,004 fresh), **Savory** (9,465 fresh), **Star Anise** (11,300), **Tarragon** (15,542 fresh), **Thyme** (157,380 dried, 27,426 fresh), **Turmeric** (127,068 dried), **Vanilla Bean Spice** (122,400 dried), **Yellow Mustard Seed** (29,257)[34] Obviously no one sits down to eat a bowl of Clove Powder, but just 2 grams (approximately one level teaspoon) added to any soup, stew, casserole, etc, brings the antioxidant power of nearly TWO POUNDS of raw carrots.

43. DIETARY FIBER (25g) – Dietary Fiber is water-soluble and supports intestinal health and also bonds to cholesterol preventing its absorption in the digestive tract. A low Fiber diet can cause digestive difficulties and increase the risk of digestive tract disease including cancer especially colon cancer which is definitely on the rise likely due to poor diet low in Dietary Fiber.[205]

FOOD	%/cal	%/g	Cals	Amt.
Pumpkin (canned)	0.337	0.115	296.4	28%
Black beans (canned)	0.303	0.274	330.3	66%
Lentils (cooked)	0.274	0.317	365.1	63%
Green Peas (canned)	0.254	0.176	393.3	30%
Fava beans (canned)	0.209	0.149	478.9	38%
Blackeye Peas (canned)	0.173	0.133	578.1	32%
Chickpeas (cooked)	0.167	0.274	597.8	45%
Lima beans (canned)	0.158	0.124	633.3	30%
Avocado	0.150	0.240	666.7	36%
Sweet Potato (naked)	0.144	0.131	692.3	26%
Dark chocolate (4oz)	0.136	0.670	736.8	76%
Wheat Germ (2.5oz)	0.120	0.423	833.3	30%
Dried Plums	0.117	0.279	853.1	49%
Pistachios	0.075	0.423	1333.3	36%
Sunflower Seed kernels	0.061	0.353	1633.3	30%
Pecans	0.055	0.388	1809.1	33%

[32][43][56][57][63][64][70][128][160][180][184][190][201][202][203][204]
Because of its well known health benefits many people are now taking Fiber from any one of a whole store isle full of products. I always recommend getting your nutrients from natural whole foods first and fiber is no exception, and it is not difficult to get if you choose the right foods. But if you are going to supplement your Dietary Fiber intake, the best source is Psyllium seed and many products are available. Avoid taking too much at one time because it is about 77% Fiber and very compact for the amount of Fiber it brings and it can definitely cause upset stomach and digestive difficulties in excess.

GETTING THE BIG 43 AND MORE

No matter what you do, it is impossible to get all of the Big 43 essential nutrients from natural whole foods on a daily basis and still stay under 2,000 calories for the day. Most people will argue that this indicates that human beings never could do it throughout our deep evolutionary past and yet they still survived. While this might be true, it does not mean that they THRIVED at all, and most scientists are certain that only in the 20th century as we began to discover the essential nutrients and learn how much of each one is needed each day did we actually "turn the corner" and improve overall health and LONGEVITY in our society.

Now that we do know a lot more than we did a hundred years ago, we are still a long way from knowing everything about the vast and complex nutritional requirements of the human body, but that does not render all that we know useless either. You must try to get the 100% RDA amounts of the following from natural whole foods: 1) The Nine Essential Amino Acids, 2) Vitamins A, B9, B12, C and K, 3) The Antioxidants, 4) Phosphorus, 5) Sulfur, 6) Fiber, 7) Potassium, 8) Sodium, 10) Chlorine, 11) Iodine, (those three are taken care of by a ½ teaspoon of SEA SALT), 12) Copper, 13) Manganese, 14) Molybdenum, and 15) Selenium.

You should make every effort to get as much as you can of the following from natural whole foods first and take supplements only to shore them up as needed: 1) Vitamins B1, B2, B3, B5, B6, D3, and E, 2) Zinc, 3) Iron, 4) The Omega-3 Fatty Acids DHA and EPA (and these Omega-3's are the ONLY ones I recommend to be supplemented regardless of how much you get from foods.)

The following may be necessary in supplement form; try to stick to low serving sizes taken throughout the day (do not take the whole daily requirement amount of any mineral especially Calcium and Magnesium all at once): 1) Vitamin B7, 2) Calcium, 3) Choline, 4) Chromium, and 5) Magnesium.

Choline and Magnesium are both very tough to get in 100% RDA amounts on a daily basis from natural whole foods and I have yet to find natural source extracts of either. The mineral products of Magnesium are harsh and should be taken in low amounts at least two to three times daily to minimize their effects.

Many natural whole plant foods bring many phytonutrients that are often unique to the food such as Pomegranates which bring a class of compounds called Punicalagins as well as Punicic Acid, and numerous studies have shown that regular consumption of Pomegranates or the juice helps lower blood pressure, improves circulation, lowers LDL cholesterol levels, lowers the risk of certain forms of cancer including breast and prostate cancer, alleviates Benign Prostate Hyperplasia, lowers the risk of heart disease, improves cognitive function and memory and can ease symptoms of arthritis. We also need as much of this healing power hidden in these foods along with the Big 43 as we can get.

You certainly don't have to do any of the math that I cover in this chapter, but it is good to know and it can be very useful in helping you to search out more foods that can provide significant nutrition and also save money.

CALCULATING NUTRIENT DENSITY

There are actually three different Nutrient Densities to consider: Amount of the nutrient per calorie, Amount of the nutrient per gram, and Amount of the nutrient per dollar cost. Many foods bring more than one essential nutrient in significant amounts. You do not need to consume 1oz of Yeast Extract Spread in order to get at least 100% of Vitamin B1 then another ounce to get the B2. So the total nutrient density is important in helping you to determine the total calories and cost that your chosen foods will incur while they provide you with their essential nutrients.

1. PERCENT PER CALORIE (%/cal) – This is the first column of each of the tables in the preceding chapter and it works like this:

1. Look up the amount in percentage of the nutrient.
2. Look up the amount of calories that amount of food has.
3. Divide the percentage by the calories.

EXAMPLE: IRON in BEEF LIVER
Since liver doesn't normally come with a nutrition label from the butcher, you can look it up either at the FDA's website which is admittedly difficult to use, or at http://nutritiondata.self.com. This page indicates that raw Beef Liver contains about 27% Iron in 100 grams which also brings about 135 calories:

27% Iron ÷ 135 calories = 0.2 %/cal of Iron

2. PERCENT PER GRAM (%/g) – For this one all you need to know is the percentage of the nutrient and the amount of grams that brings that amount of the nutrient.

1. Look up the amount in percentage of the nutrient.
2. Look up the grams of the food that brings that amount.
3. Divide the percentage by the grams.

EXAMPLE: IRON in BEEF LIVER:
Again, you can look these values up at the FDA's website or at http://nutritiondata.self.com. Using the same webpage as the first example, 100grams of Beef Liver brings 27% RDA amount of Iron:

27% Iron ÷ 100g = 0.27 %/g of Iron

3. COST PER PERCENT (¢/%) – This calculation is far more convenient if we calculate cents per percent of the nutrient in cost and you will soon see why.

1. Look up the amount in percentage of the nutrient.
2. Determine the cost of the food that brings that amount.
3. Divide the cost in cents by the percentage it provides.

EXAMPLE: IRON in BEEF LIVER:
To continue with the same food and nutrient featured in the preceding examples, 100 grams of Beef Liver brings 27% RDA

amount of Iron. Let's say that your local grocery store has fresh raw Beef Liver for sale at $3.99 per pound. Now we will need to figure out how much 100 grams of it costs. For this you will need two different numbers: 1 ounce = 28.35 grams, and 1 pound = 453.6 grams. So the question with the Beef Liver is: what fraction of 1 pound is 100 grams? And that's 100 grams/453.6 = 0.22045… which can be rounded to these four decimal places: 0.2204. Now multiply this by the cost per pound: 0.2204 x 3.99 = 0.879396. This is the price of 100 grams: $0.879396 or to the nearest cent: 88¢.

88¢ ÷ 27% Iron = 3.259¢ (cents per percent of Iron)

APPLYING THE NUTRIENT DENSITIES

The Nutrient Densities of Iron in Beef Liver are: 0.2%/cal, 0.27%/g and 3.259 cents/%. These are a bit abstract, so let's apply these numbers to answer the three big REAL WORLD questions: How many calories will it take to get 100% RDA of Iron, How much Liver is that (in ounces)? And how much will it cost?

1. HOW MANY CALORIES TO GET 100%? Divide 100 by the nutrient density in %/cal: For Iron in Beef Liver:

100 ÷ 0.2%/cal = 200 calories.

2. HOW MUCH LIVER IS THAT? Divide 100 by the nutrient density in %/g. For the Iron in Beef Liver:

100 ÷ 0.27%/g = 370.37 grams

To convert this back to ounces: Divide the amount by 28.35:

370.37 grams ÷ 28.35g/oz = 13.06 ounces

3. HOW MUCH WILL THAT AMOUNT COST? This calculation is the easiest of all. Take the nutrient density in cents per percent and just put a dollar sign in front of it.

3.259 ¢/% Iron in Beef Liver ➔ $3.259 or $3.26 to get 100% RDA amount of Iron from Beef Liver.

EVALUATING THE FOOD

.Even those who truly love Beef Liver might not want to eat 13 ounces of it (nearly a pound) per day to get their Iron. And when it comes to animal meats, there are two additional important factors to consider: Saturated Fat and Cholesterol. For plant foods, some also bring Fats and the other consideration is the "Carb Load" (the amount of simple sugars and starches the food brings.) While at the webpage that provided the data (or if it is included in the food's Nutrition Label) the amount of Saturated Fat, Cholesterol and Carbohydrates is also available. On the webpage switch the amount of the food to 1 ounce. This reveals that 1 ounce of Beef Liver contains: 2% Saturated Fat and 26% Cholesterol. Multiply each of these by 13 (ounces) that we determined is necessary to get 100% RDA amount of Iron for the day:

2% Saturated Fat/oz x 13 ounces = 26% Saturated Fat

26% Cholesterol/oz x 13 ounces = 338% Cholesterol

And that is an outrageous and indeed DANGEROUS amount of Cholesterol which means, not only is the Liver going to cost you about $3.26 per day to get the Iron you need ($3.26 x 30 = $97.80

per month) it is also going to clog your arteries with far too much cholesterol making it an unhealthy and impractical source of Iron. It is certainly alright to consume 3 ounces of it once in a while and to count that Iron for the day (about 23%) but other sources would be necessary to complete the 100% amount for that day.

MORE NUTRIENT DENSITY EXAMPLES

Now let's try plain old cabbage. It is one of my favorite foods and also one of my favorite examples for calculating nutrient densities.

EXAMPLE: VITAMIN C in BOILED CABBAGE

Values obtained from http://nutritiondata.self.com:
100g has 62% Vitamin C and 23 calories:

62% ÷ 23 cal = 2.695 %/cal of Vitamin C

62% ÷ 100g = 0.62 %/g of Vitamin C

The local grocery store sells Cabbage for 69¢ per pound:

100/453.6 = 0.2204 x 69¢ = 15.2¢

15.2¢ ÷ 62% = 0.245 ¢/%

Calories to get 100%:

100 ÷ 2.695 %/cal = 37.1 calories.

How much Cabbage is that?

100 ÷ 0.62 %/g = 161.29 grams

161.29 grams ÷ 28.35g/oz = 5.69 ounces

How much does that amount cost?

0.245 ¢/% ➔ $0.245 = 24 ½ cents

Evaluation: Total Fats = 0, Starches = 0, Sugars = 2.8g/100g. Cabbage is very low calorie and has a "Carb Load" of just 2.8% sugars and starches by weight which is very low. Just 24 ½ cents per day, $7.35 per month ($0.245 x 30,) will cover 100% RDA of Vitamin C. The same amount, 100 grams, of Cabbage also brings 136% Vitamin K which means the 5.7 ounces has over double the amount of Vitamin K (over 200%) as well. Since a reasonable portion size can inexpensively cover two essential nutrients, for very few calories, Cabbage is an excellent affordable Functional Food.

EXAMPLE: VITAMIN A in COD LIVER OIL

Values obtained from http://nutritiondata.self.com:
1 Teaspoon is 4 grams and contains 90% Vitamin A and 40.6 calories

90% ÷ 40.6 cal = 2.216 %/cal of Vitamin A

90% ÷ 4g = 22.5 %/g of Vitamin A

The local grocery store sells Cod Liver Oil for $4.99 for a 10oz (310g) bottle. In this case we know the exact weight of the amount being consumed and the exact weight of the whole product. Therefore we divide the amount of the serving by the total weight of the product then multiply by the price:

4/310 = 0.0129 x 499 cents = 6.347¢

6.347¢ ÷ 90% = 0.071 ¢/%

Because the amounts are small here, we will just use the cost of the teaspoonful which is 6.347 cents to get 90% RDA amount of Vitamin A each day.

Calories to get 100%:

$100 \div 2.216$ %/cal = 45.1 calories.

How much Cod Liver Oil is that?

$100 \div 22.5$ %/g = 4.44 grams

(A little more than the teaspoonful which was expected.)

How much does that amount cost?

0.071 ¢/% ➔ $0.071 = 7.1 cents

EVALUATION: Since each teaspoonful brings 90% RDA which is very good and costs 6.347 cents, it costs 6.347 x 30 = $1.90 per month (less than the bottle, so it will last over two months.) The data on the webpage indicates that the teaspoonful also brings 113% RDA of Vitamin D3 and 888mg Omega-3 Fatty Acids (DHA and EPA) and 5% of the Daily Limit of Saturated Fat and 8% of the Daily Limit of Cholesterol. The oil is very high in both of these but you only need to take the teaspoon so these values are tolerable. Since it is so inexpensive and brings four of the Big 43 – Vitamin A, Vitamin D3 and the Omega-3 Fatty Acids DHA and EPA, this is a very inexpensive and effective "Functional Food" or it is better to call it a natural supplement.

EXAMPLE: VITAMIN A in a RAW CARROT

Each carrot has a different size, so we'll use the average from a 2 pound bag. Values obtained from http://nutritiondata.self.com: 100 grams brings 41.0 calories and 334% Vitamin A as beta-Carotene.

$334\% \div 41.0$ cal = 8.146 %/cal of Vitamin A

$334\% \div 100g$ = 3.34 %/g of Vitamin A

The local grocery store sells the bag for $1.99, that's $1 per pound:

$100/453.6 = 0.2204$ x 100 cents = 22.04¢

22.04¢ $\div$ 334% = 0.0659 ¢/%

Calories to get 100%:

$100 \div 8.146$ %/cal = 12.27 calories.

How much Raw Carrot is that?

$100 \div 3.34$ %/g = 29.94 grams

$29.94g \div 28.35$ g/oz = 1.056 ounces

How much does that amount cost?

0.0659 ¢/% ➔ $0.0659 = 6.59 cents

A sample bag contained 14 carrots and weighed 2 pounds or 32 ounces:

32 ounces $\div$ 14 carrots = 2.28 ounces each

EVALUATION: Roughly half of one carrot will weigh more than 1.056 ounces and bring over 100% RDA amount of Vitamin A as beta-Carotene. There are 14 carrots in the bag times 2 yields 28 halves that cost $1.99: 199 cents divided by 28 = 7.1 cents per day x 30 = $2.13 cents per month. 100 grams of Raw Carrots contain: Saturated Fat = 0, Cholesterol = 0, Starches = 1.4g and Sugars = 4.7g; 1.4 + 4.7 = 6.1g per 100g so the "Carb Load" is 6.1% which is very good. Carrots are a very inexpensive and healthy way to get plenty of Vitamin A and have one of the highest nutrient densities in terms of percent of Vitamin A per Calorie of any food.

ANTIOXIDANT ORAC DENSITY

I often make a point that a given food has the antioxidant power of a certain number of pounds of raw carrots. It is important to realize that each antioxidant is unique. Each has its own affinities – which oxidants they are good at neutralizing in the body (and there are many different oxidants) and each one has a different potential – how many of these oxidants it can neutralize before being used up (actual numbers of molecules of oxidants that a given amount of the antioxidant can neutralize.) Furthermore, different organs in the body have their own affinities for which antioxidants they like to absorb. All cells essentially like all antioxidants, but each organ has its favorites that it will greedily soak up when they are present in the blood stream. Since they all behave in so many different ways it is impossible for any measurement to truly reflect their antioxidant potential side-by-side. While the ORAC (Oxygen Radical Absorption Capacity) score for foods is now considered obsolete, it is really no better or worse than any other method of comparing any two foods side-by-side.

ANTIOXIDANT POWER VERSUS RAW CARROTS

This calculation is an easy eye-opener to do. Since all foods are tested with the same amount (100 grams) then they all basically sit side-by-side. But when we want to compare different amounts of the foods, that's when we need to do a little math.

EXAMPLE: OREGANO versus RAW CARROTS

For all dried spices we will assume that 1 teaspoon weighs 2 grams. Therefore if 1 teaspoon of dried Oregano has an ORAC Score of 175,295 and raw Carrots have an ORAC score of 697:

175,295 ÷ 697 = 251.499… or 251.5

This is how much stronger the Oregano is gram for gram. So 2 grams will provide the antioxidant power of:

251.5 x 2 grams = 503 grams of raw Carrots

Convert to ounces:

503 grams ÷ 28.35 grams/ounce = 17.74 ounces

So 1 teaspoon of dried Oregano has the antioxidant ORAC power of almost 18 ounces of Raw Carrots. Putting that teaspoon of Oregano into your lunch soup is like dumping over a pound of raw carrots into it in terms of the antioxidant power it will bring.

ORAC DENSITY

In this calculation we want to compare the antioxidant power a food provides versus the calories in brings. The Top 50 Foods based on their Antioxidant Density per calorie are provided in the preceding chapter and this is how the calculation is done.

EXAMPLE: PECANS versus RAW CARROTS

This is a good pair of foods to compare because the Carrots are a Net Negative Calorie food at about 10.1 cal/ounce, but Pecans are loaded with Fat and bring about 199 cal/ounce. The question then becomes; for the same amount of antioxidant power, which will cost you more in calories, Pecans or Carrots?

1. Determine the power of the same weight of Pecans versus Carrots:

   17,940 (Pecans ORAC score) ÷ 697 (Carrots score) = 25.738

2. Determine the ratio of calories of Pecans to Carrots:

   199cal/oz (Pecans) ÷ 10.1 cal/oz (Carrots) = 19.70

CONCLUSION: Although Pecans bring a lot more calories, 19.7 times as much for any given amount, they still bring 25.74 times as many antioxidants and are the better choice.

ORAC DENSITY PER CALORIE

EXAMPLE: PECANS

Pecans have an ORAC score of 17,940 determined with 100 grams therefore:

   100g ÷ 28.35 grams/ounce = 3.527 ounces

   3.527oz x 199cal/oz = 701.873 calories

Therefore, 701.873 calories deliver an ORAC score of 17,940:

   17,940 ÷ 701.873 = 25.560 ORAC per Calorie

The higher this number is, then the more antioxidant power you get per calorie.

EXAMPLE: RAW CARROTS

Raw Carrots have an ORAC score of 697 determined with 100g:

   100g ÷ 28.35 grams/ounce = 3.527 ounces

   3.527oz x 10.1cal/oz = 35.6227 calories

Therefore, 35.6227 calories deliver an ORAC score of 697:

   697 ÷ 35.6227 = 19.566 ORAC per Calorie

APPLYING THE ORAC DENSITIES

EXAMPLE: How much raw Carrot and how many calories of them will it take to equal the antioxidant power of 2 ounces of Pecans?

   17,940 (Pecans ORAC score) ÷ 697 (Carrots score) = 25.738

Ounce for ounce it will take 25.738 times as much raw Carrots to equal the antioxidants delivered by Pecans:

   2 ounces (Pecans) x 25.738 = 51.476 ounces Raw Carrots

   51.476 ounces x 10.1 cal/oz = 519.9076

For Raw Carrots to deliver the same Oxygen Radical Absorption Capacity of 2 ounces of Pecans you would need to eat 51.5 oz (3 ¼ pounds) and that would bring almost 520 calories while the 2 ounces of Pecans "only" bring 398 calories. However, each plant does bring different antioxidants, so you shouldn't think about replacing one food with another, but instead look for foods with high antioxidant content to ADD to your daily diet; the more different antioxidants you take in, the more chances are that all of them will find their way into all of the organ systems in your body and provide their "oxidative relief" and improve your health.

It is important to understand that losing weight is hard to do. I tried many different diets based on commercial packaged food products and was disappointed by them all until I realized why they all fail: they don't directly address the problem. And the problem is not as simple as dramatically reducing your caloric intake.

Whenever you do this – go from consuming well over 2,000 calories per day, to suddenly consuming far fewer than 2,000 calories per day – several things hit you all at the same time. 1) Your body is accustomed to receiving all of those extra calories and when they disappear, you feel hungry all day long. 2) Your nutritional intake will also radically change and your body will immediately crave the nutrients in the foods that you were eating before you changed your daily eating regimen. 3) By drastically and suddenly reducing your caloric intake, the body goes into "famine shock" mode; it begins to produce Cortisol and a host of other hormones and chemical changes which discourage the adipose (fat) cells from releasing their stores of fat, and also depress the metabolism to conserve energy.

The net result of all of this is that a person who tries to "go on a diet" is immediately hit with miserable hunger and cravings as well as a depressed metabolism which in turn causes lethargy, fatigue, and wreaks havoc on brain function causing mental issues such as depression, anxiety, etc. It is certainly not as bad as trying to go cold turkey from harsh narcotics, but that is no consolation for anyone suffering these very real and very miserable effects.

Personally, I was willing to "tough it out" and go through all of that misery in order to lose the weight, but every time I tried, within a week I had GAINED weight while starving on the limited calories of the major "diet plans" and their tasteless foods in small portions. At that point I gave up. Why bother suffering to lose weight when all I ever got for my trouble was weight GAIN?

The answer is to combat the body's effort to conserve energy while the calories are limited. Do not underestimate the power of the holistic herbs. And do not get discouraged if at first they don't work for you. Some are stronger than others (which can also make long-term usage of them dangerous) and each one has a unique set of phytonutrients; two different plants with the same property such as "Diuretic" (prevents water retention) likely have different naturally occurring chemicals and one might work very well on you while the other will not. Others may take a few days to take effect because they have an effect similar to steroids; in fact, many of them are steroids. Just bear in mind that these are nothing like the steroids with the evil reputations in sports. This term means that they act like hormones so they trigger cells to alter their internal metabolic functions rather than directly take action, and it is those changes to the cells that over time will result in the positive effect you want.

THE DIURETICS – FIGHTING WATER RETENTION

The diuretics cause the kidneys to absorb water out of the blood stream and eliminate it. As this happens all of the tissues in the body must begin to release water back into the bloodstream to compensate which can lead to symptoms of dehydration which is very harsh on all organ systems especially the brain. In fact, hangovers are primarily the result of dehydration caused by the severe diuretic effect of alcohol. Beer is even stronger because of the Hops which like many of the following holistic herbs and foods are also diuretic in nature.

There are plenty more plants in my database that are noted for being diuretics than those in the following list. However, I have only included those that are well known and often prescribed for their diuretic power. If not, then it is fair to say that while a plant might actually have this property, it is probably not as prominent as its other properties and we want strong, effective diuretics.

As long as you are drinking plenty of clear liquids and the best of course is pure drinking water, then usage of diuretics is a good course of action if you do suffer from water retention. Diuretics help the kidneys by encouraging them not only to absorb water from the bloodstream and remove it, but this also helps flush their intricate structures and encourages them to remove other waste products from the blood as well. Do not overdo it with the diuretics and if you have or even suspect that you might have weak or overworked kidneys or kidney disease, CHECK WITH A DOCTOR BEFORE USING THESE MEDICINAL HERBS. Some are quite potent and can put a DANGEROUS strain on the kidneys if they are already weak. And if you aren't even aware that your kidneys are weak, you could suffer sudden KIDNEY FAILURE.

1. BEARBERRY (Arctostaphylos uva-ursi) – A.k.a. Uva-ursi is well known for usage in Urinary Tract Infections and is also a strong diuretic. Do not use if you have kidney disease or weak or overworked kidneys.[39]

RECOMMENDED BEARBERRY LEAF SUPPLEMENT
===
MANUFACTURER: SWANSON VITAMINS
PRODUCT NAME: PREMIUM UVA URSI CAPSULES
WEBSITE: www. swansonvitamins.com
PRODUCT PAGE: https://www.swansonvitamins.com/
swanson-premium-uva-ursi-leaf-450-mg-100-caps
Swanson Vitamins produces reasonable quality supplements in terms of ingredients and manufacturing quality, are they are superior to most store-bought brands. And they do carry many of these lesser known holistic herb supplements at very reasonable prices. Swanson is the only source I could find for many of the holistic herbs included in these lists.

2. BLACK PEPPER (Piper nigrum) – The health benefits of plain black pepper are incredible. It is a compound called Piperine which gives it that distinctive aroma, flavor, and ability to irritate the nasal cavity and make you sneeze. Piperine has been shown in many studies to aid digestion by activating all digestive fluids production from the salivary glands, to the stomach lining to the intestinal walls where it not only stimulates the production of the digestive enzymes but also enhances cellular membrane permeability. That is a fancy way of saying that it allows the surface cells in the intestines to absorb all nutrients in the meal more readily, so you get more nutrients out of the entire meal particularly fats and other large molecules that are normally difficult to absorb and digest. As long as you are eating foods that are low in fat, this is actually a very good thing because breaking them down yields other useful molecules that will not necessarily be stored again as fat, but rather get used for other jobs or right away as fuel. It also helps with the absorption of nutrients that are oil (or fat) soluble like Vitamin E. Piperine has been shown in at least one scientific study to selectively target and kill at least one form of colon cancer cells while helping all of the healthy cells in the colon. Finally, Black Pepper is a diuretic that can stimulate the kidneys to pull water from the bloodstream and eliminate it. Piperine is very volatile so ground black pepper has lost a lot of its punch; freshly ground whole peppercorns applied with a grinder to food as it is served is the best way to get in on its many excellent health benefits.[40]

3. BUCHU (Agathosma betulina) – This is a very strong, proven diuretic herb that is actually the main ingredient of two OTC (Over The Counter) drugs: Fluidex and Odrinil (used as premenstrual diuretics, but water retention is NOT limited to women, many men suffer from it as well, they just don't notice it like women do.) This use in medications proves that many of these holistic herbs do have REAL power and they are not nonsense at all. Buchu has a long history of use in southern Africa (its native range) and is still made into tinctures in Europe to treat hangovers, cold/flu, etc. Dietary supplements and bulk dried leaf, said to have a mint-like aroma should be easy to find. Follow the directions and go easy on it because BUCHU SHOULD NOT BE USED BY FOLKS WITH KIDNEY PROBLEMS.[41]

RECOMMENDED BUCHU LEAF SUPPLEMENT
==
MANUFACTURER: SWANSON VITAMINS
PRODUCT NAME: PREMIUM BUCHU LEAF EXTRACT
WEBSITE: www. swansonvitamins.com
PRODUCT PAGE: https://www.swansonvitamins.com/ swanson-premium-full-spectrum-buchu-leaf-4-1-extract-100-mg-60-caps

4. BUTCHER'S BROOM (Ruscus aculeatus) – Also called Jew's Myrtle, has a long history of usage as an effective diuretic and as a blood vessel toner. The German Commission E has approved its internal usage for "venous insufficiency" and it is a popular natural holistic treatment for varicose veins and hemorrhoids (usually caused by poor circulation, by the way.) Butcher's Broom comes highly recommended and can be found in supplements as well as bulk dried powdered root forms.[80]

TOP RECOMMENDED BUTCHER'S BROOM SUPPLEMENT

MANUFACTURER: NOW FOODS
PRODUCT NAME: BUTCHER'S BROOM CAPSULES
WEBSITE: www.nowfoods.com
PRODUCT PAGE: www.nowfoods.com/supplements/
butchers-broom-capsules

5. CELERY (Apium graviolens) – Celery is one of nature's true power tools. It contains high concentrations of both Apiole and Apigenin, two phytoestrogens that can help with women's health issues linked to Estrogen imbalance. But it is not just for women. It also helps with blood vessel toning and is a strong diuretic. Fresh stalks, or cooked into soups and stews as well as the powdered seed used as a spice can help with many issues including: reduce water retention, improve circulation, provide those phytoestrogens (men benefit from them as well), and serve as an excellent Net Negative Calorie food for losing weight.[81]

6. CHANCA PIEDRA (Phyllanthus niruri) – This is one of the strongest holistic herbs known to science and CAUTION in its usage is STRONGLY ADVISED. The plant has been used by Central and South American natives for centuries to cure kidney stones and it is highly effective. IF YOU HAVE OR SUSPECT YOU HAVE KIDNEY OR URINARY TRACT STONES, SEE A DOCTOR. Scientists have also found active compounds that may be potent antivirals for treating Hepatitis B and HIV. They have also found that it contains Aldose Reductase inhibitors that may help stop nerve damage. It also happens to be a strong diuretic as well. For casual use as a diuretic you should take it no more than once every three to five days. Again, it is very powerful and IF YOU HAVE WEAK KIDNEYS OR KIDNEY DISEASE, CHECK WITH YOUR DOCTOR BEFORE USING CHANCE PIEDRA.[83]

TOP RECOMMENDED CHANCA PIEDRA PRODUCT

MANUFACTURER: SunFood
PRODUCT NAME: Wild-Crafted Chanca Piedra Herbal Tea
VENDOR WEBSITE: www.vitacost.com

Make a batch of the herbal tea as directed and only drink about one fourth of the recommended amount every three to five days.

7. CLEAVERS (Galium aparine) – This is a Top Recommended Holistic Herb and well known for its diuretic power. All members of the genus Galium have strong pleasant aromas. Sweet Woodruff (G. odoratum) is used in some perfumes. Young leaves are edible like spinach and the seeds are roasted and used to make a coffee substitute. The point is that this is a safe edible plant and it is well known in herbalism as a diuretic, depurative (detoxifies the blood and bodily tissues by directly assisting the lymphatic system,) treats Urinary Tract Infections, and lowers blood pressure without affecting heart rate. Cleavers is not easy to find in supplement form, but bulk dried leaf is available online and can be made into herbal tea. Fresh is far better and live plants and seeds are also available.[82]

RECOMMENDED CLEAVERS PRODUCT
==

MANUFACTURER: Celebration Herbals
PRODUCT NAME: Cleavers Herb Bulk Tea
VENDOR WEBSITE: www.vitacost.com
PRODUCT PAGE: https://www.vitacost.com/celebration-herbals-cleavers-herb-bulk-tea-caffeine-free

8. CORIANDER and CILANTRO (Coriandrum sativum) –
Coriander is a Top Recommended Spice and is the ground seeds of the same plant as Cilantro which is the fresh or dried leaves. Both are diuretics and very safe to use. While both are effective, the seeds are much stronger. Coriander is also a well known anti-inflammatory. In conjunction with other immune system boosters like Garlic and the Omega-3 Fatty Acids it has been shown to cure chronic infections. You can make your own herbal tea from the fresh or dried leaf Cilantro or from the powdered Coriander.[89]

9. CRANBERRY (Vaccinium macrocarpa) – This relative of the Blueberry has the highest antioxidant power per calorie of any readily available food and has been shown in numerous studies to reduce cardiovascular disease, diabetes, urinary tract infections and tooth decay. Its power comes from unique compounds that prevent bacteria from sticking to the tissues that they are invading allowing them to be flushed away. It is also a strong diuretic and 100% pure Cranberry juice is low calorie, outstanding for your overall health, and safe in moderation.[76]

10. CUMIN (Cuminum cyminum) – This is a Top Recommended Spice. It adds a wonderful hearty flavor to beef and ground turkey and aside from being a diuretic; it promotes digestion and is used for various stomach complaints. Modern science is studying Cumin seed's anticancer properties too so dust off the old spice rack and start putting those powerful medicinal plants to work for you.[77]

11. DANDELION (Taraxacum officinale) – The health benefits of Dandelion Root are legendary and well deserved. It is a potent depurative especially for liver health and can promote healthy skin and reduce acne by reducing the amount of Androgen in the body which aggravates acne. Its potent depurative and diuretic action has earned it a place in some herbal weight-loss products and studies have shown that it does help people lose weight. Products abound on the market. It is potent medicine so use it sparingly.[78]

TOP RECOMMENDED DANDELION SUPPLEMENT
==

MANUFACTURER: NOW FOODS
PRODUCT NAME: Dandelion Root 500 mg Capsules
WEBSITE: www.nowfoods.com
PRODUCT PAGE: www.nowfoods.com/supplements/
dandelion-root-500-mg-capsules

12. HORSETAIL (Equisetum arvense) – Horsetail's primary historical use in holism is as a diuretic making it one of the better choices in the list. It is most often used as an herbal tea which must be boiled for about 3 hours to extract the active compounds from this tough grass. Not for use by those with weak kidneys, kidney disease, kidney stones or those on blood pressure medication containing ACE (Angiotensin Converting Enzyme) inhibitors. Drink plenty of water when using it.[79]

TOP RECOMMENDED HORSETAIL SUPPLEMENT
==

MANUFACTURER: NATURE'S WAY
PRODUCT NAME: Horsetail Grass 440mg Capsules
VENDOR WEBSITE: www.naturesway.com

The current hype surrounding Horsetail has to do with bone and joint health and this might be true, but it is definitely a diuretic.

13. JUNIPER BERRY (Juniperus communis) – Herbal tea made from the dried fruit is a potent diuretic and caution is advised in making the herbal tea. The essential oil is for external use only. Do not use if you have weak or diseased kidneys. JUNIPER BERRY IS NOT FOR DAILY LONG-TERM USE WHICH CAN LEAD TO KIDNEY PROBLEMS.[84]

RECOMMENDED JUNIPER BERRY SUPPLEMENT
==

MANUFACTURER: SWANSON VITAMINS
PRODUCT NAME: PREMIUM JUNIPER BERRIES
WEBSITE: www. swansonvitamins.com
PRODUCT PAGE: https://www.swansonvitamins.com/
swanson-premium-juniper-berries-520-mg-100-caps

Despite the name, the product is capsules, not whole berries.

14. LAVENDER (Lavandula spp.) – Lavender is best known for the calming effect of its essential oil especially in aromatherapy, but the whole above ground plant is actually edible. It has been approved for internal use by the German Commission E for high blood pressure, nervous stomach issues and insomnia. Lavender improves circulation and is strong medicine for skin ailments. It is also a mild diuretic, Below is the only internal supplement I could find.[85]

TOP RECOMMENDED LAVENDER SUPPLEMENT
==

MANUFACTURER: Integrative Therapeutics
PRODUCT NAME: Lavela WS 1265

VENDOR WEBSITE: www.integrativepro.com/products/
neuroendocrine/lavela-ws-1265

15. LOVAGE (Levisticum officinale) – A popular English garden
herb for centuries, this close relative to Celery has many similar
properties and is best known as a diuretic and is relatively safe.
Supplements may be very difficult to find, but viable seeds can be
found for those who wish to grow their own.[87]

16. MOTHERWORT (Leonurus cardica) – In Traditional Chinese
Medicine this is considered a longevity tonic and a heart tonic.
Motherwort improves circulation, lowers blood pressure and lowers
heart rate. Because of this last effect it should be not be used
daily. It is also a strong diuretic that reduces inflammation and
swelling which also improves blood pressure.[90]

RECOMMENDED MOTHERWORT SUPPLEMENT
===

MANUFACTURER: SWANSON VITAMINS
PRODUCT NAME: FULL SPECTRUM MOTHERWORT
WEBSITE: www. swansonvitamins.com
PRODUCT PAGE: www.swansonvitamins.com/swanson-
premium-full-spectrum-motherwort-400-mg-60-caps

IF YOU ARE ON CURRENTLY ANY LONG-TERM MEDICATION
ESPECIALLY HEART, HIGH BLOOD PRESSURE, OR BLOOD
THINNER MEDICATIONS, OR HAVE KIDNEY ISSUES, DO NOT
USE MOTHERWORT. ASK YOUR DOCTOR BEFORE USING
MOTHERWORT.

17. PARSLEY (Petroselinum crispum) – Parsley is so commonly
used in the culinary arts that most folks are unaware of its holistic
power. Parsley is a potent diuretic and you can make herbal tea
from the dried leaf parsley flakes but, don't overdo it (once every
few days) because it does contain Calcium Oxalate crystals which
can lead to kidney or gallbladder stones. The tea is quite bitter and
aids digestion and due to trace mineral content like Boron may
also improve bone health. You can flavor the tea with Lemon (or
Lime) juice and fresh Stevia leaf (both also in these lists) both of
which also bring potent health benefits.[91]

18. PLANTAIN (Plantago major) – Not to be confused with the
large starchy bananas with the same name, this is a small weed-
like herb with big health benefits. The whole plant, roots and all,
can be thoroughly washed of soil and dropped in the blender with
warm water. It will turn into a dark green thick soup which can be
stored for a week or two. Plantain, or Ribwort if you prefer, aside
from being a good depurative and diuretic is also a styptic that can
stop the bleeding of small cuts and is also used on bee stings.[92]

RECOMMENDED PLANTAIN SUPPLEMENT
===

MANUFACTURER: SWANSON VITAMINS
PRODUCT NAME: FULL SPECTRUM PLANTAIN LEAF
WEBSITE: www. swansonvitamins.com

PRODUCT PAGE: www.swansonvitamins.com/swanson-premium-full-spectrum-plantain-leaf-plantago-major-400-mg-60-caps

19. REHMANNIA (Rehmannia glutinosa) – Chinese Foxglove has a long history of usage in Traditional Chinese Medicine and has many uses: lower back pain due to kidney issues (it restores vitality to the kidneys), cough, fever, diabetes, deafness, urinary incontinence, uterine bleeding, vertigo, tinnitus, regulation of menstrual flow, and chronic fatigue. Rehmannia root also protects and supports the liver as well as the adrenal glands. Finally, it is a depurative and a diuretic. Rehmannia is available in supplement form as well as dried bulk powder. This is the only true Kidney Tonic that helps revitalize the kidneys in this entire list (although there are reports that Celery has the same property, if to a lesser extent) and I highly recommend it.[93]

TOP RECOMMENDED REHMANNIA SUPPLEMENT
==

SOURCE: LUCKY VITAMINS
PRODUCT NAME: Rehmannia Endurance 837mg
VENDOR WEBSITE: https://www.luckyvitamin.com/p-4283-planetary-herbals-rehmannia-endurance-837-mg-150-tablets-formerly-planetary-formulas

IF YOU HAVE WEAK, OVERWORKED, OR DISEASED KIDNEYS ASK YOUR DOCTOR BEFORE USING REHMANNIA. USE THIS HERB SPARINGLY – IT IS STRONG MEDICINE.

20. ROSEMARY (Rosmarinus officinalis) – This is another plant that makes my Top Recommended Spices and for good reason. Rosemary has one of the longest lists of medicinal properties and is used to treat more afflictions than any other herb in this list. While it is best known for its effect on the Central Nervous System to improve circulation, it is also considered a heart tonic. It also improves oxygen transfer across the blood-brain barrier and some studies have shown that it improves concentration and memory. It is also both a diuretic and a diaphoretic (promotes detoxification of the body through sweating) and is an excellent choice for any dish but especially those that take longer to cook like roasts and slow cooked stews.[94]

21. STINGING NETTLE (Urtica dioica) – Although the fresh raw plant is covered in fine hair-like thorns that induce a painful itching and burning rash on contact, the plant can be soaked in water which dissolves these irritating hairs and results in leaves and young stalks that are edible raw or cooked. While the hairs contain histamine, the same active compound in bee stings, the rest of the plant contains very strong antihistamines (likely to protect itself from its own defenses) and it is used for treating asthma and other chronic allergies. It is a potent diuretic and safe to eat or make herbal tea AFTER you have given it a long soak and tossed that water out.[95]

RECOMMENDED STINGING NETTLE SUPPLEMENT

===

MANUFACTURER: SWANSON VITAMINS
PRODUCT NAME: PREMIUM STINGING NETTLE ROOT
WEBSITE: www. swansonvitamins.com
PRODUCT PAGE: www.swansonvitamins.com/swanson-premium-stinging-nettle-root-500-mg-100-caps
The root is allegedly stronger medicine than the leaves.

22. WATERCRESS (Nasturtium officinale) – This is one of the very best "Functional Foods" on the planet. Despite being very low calorie, it has the second highest nutrient density of Vitamin C, and it is also a powerful diuretic. Watercress, Celery, Bean sprouts, Onions and chopped green Cabbage can form the foundation for a wonderful Chow Mein (clear stew) for lean chicken breast.[97]

CONCLUSION

There are plenty of potent diuretics to choose from, both as supplements as well as edible vegetables and spices that can certainly help alleviate water retention. I use most of the edibles and spices on a regular basis in my diet and you should too. Just be very sure that you DO NOT HAVE KIDNEY PROBLEMS before you jump into the deep end and include too many of them all at once. Those who do not get regular doctor checkups and plan to begin a SERIOUS DIET intended to lose weight and suffer from water retention and plan to take some of the stronger herbs in this list MUST get a checkup first and inform your doctor that you plan to start a healthy Natural Whole Foods and Holistic Herbs Diet and that you want to be checked for any sign of KIDNEY PROBLEMS. Because Celery has at least one study showing that it has kidney protective properties and Rehmannia is also a verified restorative for the kidneys, these two are the best ones to add to your effort along with the other edible foods and spices.

These plants are essential to the task at hand: losing unwanted pounds. Aside from increasing your "get up and go," this causes a welcome side effect of making you feel better with that additional spring in your step. The increased metabolism and energy they provide means that they are stimulating the body to burn more fuel and if your caloric intake has gone way down through a liberal usage of the Net Negative Calorie foods, then these holistic plants will force your body to dip into the fat reserves and burn them; and that is exactly what anyone on a diet needs. Some of these are stimulants, others contain compounds like Synephrine found in Grapefruit which dial up your metabolism and encourage the body to burn away excess stored calories held in fat tissue.

INCREASED ENERGY/METABOLISM PLANTS

1. AÇAI (Euterpe oleracea) – Despite the hype, Açai is loaded with anthocyanidins, powerful antioxidants, and has a reputation for increasing the metabolism and helping with weight loss. There are plenty of products, but the 100% Pure Juice is the best way to get in on the health benefits. The Recommended product is about 94% and contains no chemical additives.[98]

RECOMMENDED ACAI PEODUCT

==

MANUFACTURER: ZOLA
PRODUCT NAME: ORGANIC ACAI JUICE 32oz
VENDOR WEBSITE: www.vitacost.com
PRODUCT PAGE: https://www.vitacost.com/zola-organic-acai-juice-original-32-fl-oz-1

2. BANABA (Lagerstroemia speciosa) – This plant is also starting to show up in many herbal weight-loss supplements and contains a verified metabolic stimulant called Corosolic Acid.[101]

RECOMMENDED BANABA SUPPLEMENT

==

MANUFACTURER: SWANSON VITAMINS
PRODUCT NAME: HIGH POTENCY BANABA EXTRACT
WEBSITE: www. swansonvitamins.com
PRODUCT PAGE: www.swansonvitamins.com/swanson-superior-herbs-high-potency-banaba-extract-2-corosolic-acid-60-mg-90-caps

BANABA IS VERY STRONG, USE IT IN MODERATION. BANABA IS NOT FOR LONG-TERM DAILY USE.

3. BITTER MELON (Momordica charantia) – This relative of the cucumber despite having a bitter taste is a popular vegetable in many countries. Long-term overindulgence is not recommended and has been linked to serious health issues. This vegetable's unique and powerful triterpenoids have been shown to reduce adipose (fat) cell formation and they also stimulate the burning of stored fat.[100]

4. BLACK PEPPER (Piper nigrum) – All members of the genus including Long Pepper (P. longum) Java Pepper (P. retrofractum) etc, contain Piperine amongst other phytonutrients that promote digestion by helping the intestines to absorb all nutrients in the meal, and they also increase metabolism. Also featured in the preceding list as a diuretic, it should come as no surprise that Black Pepper is one of my Top Recommended Spices and a mainstay in a healthy diet.[40]

5. CINNAMON (Cinnamomum zeylanicum, C. cassia) – The health benefits of Cinnamon are truly amazing. It has the ability to assist in blood sugar regulation and insulin pathways and it is considered a powerful medicinal herb for the prevention and even treatment of Type II diabetes. It also activates the metabolism and can help with weight loss. Store bought cinnamon powder is a bit old and stale and has lost a lot of its medicinal potency, but you can grind the sticks yourself and get a lot more powerful punch. Cinnamon is considered relatively safe but it is a strong astringent (promotes water retention) and rubifacient (contact irritant.) The oil is very strong so overindulgence of the oil is not recommended. Supplement products abound but avoid all products that have added the artificial chemical Chromium picolinate because some health professionals believe that this is a possible cancer causing agent.[86]

TOP RECOMMENDED CINNAMON SUPPLEMENT
==

MANUFACTURER: NOW FOODS
PRODUCT NAME: CINNAMON BARK 500MG ORGANIC
WEBSITE: www.nowfoods.com
PRODUCT PAGE: www.nowfoods.com/supplements/
cinnamon-bark-500-mg-organic

6. CORIANDER and CILANTRO (Coriandrum sativum) – Prized as a culinary spice, Cilantro is a powerful herb that helps the body detoxify and can help mitigate metal poisoning especially in the liver. It also enhances the metabolism and can help with weight loss. The ground seeds are also a spice called Coriander which also has remarkable health benefits and is in the preceding list of Diuretics, but it is somewhat bitter. Both can be used in soups, salad dressing, stews, casseroles, and even herbal teas.[89]

7. COCONUT (Cocos nucifera) – Coconut stimulates energy metabolism, lowers cholesterol and balances hormonal levels. You get a whole host of benefits from this amazing functional food. Coconut milk, pulp, and extra virgin oil are all loaded with high quantities of some relatively rare phytonutrients called Medium Chain Triglycerides that bring all of these benefits.[104]

TOP RECOMMENDED COCONUT OIL PRODUCT
==

MANUFACTURER: JARROW FORMULAS

PRODUCT NAME: ORGANIC COCONUT OIL 32oz.
VENDOR WEBSITE: www.vitacost.com
PRODUCT PAGE: www.vitacost.com/jarrow-formulas-organic-coconut-oil-32-fl-oz

Refined Coconut Oil also sold as "neutral" (no flavor) is what you will find in most grocery stores and is NOT a good form. This recommended product may be expensive but it is cold expeller pressed (Virgin and unrefined) and organic (no chemicals used in the growth of the trees) and is well worth it.

8. COFFEE (Coffea arabica) – This is the second most heavily abused plant consumed by people worldwide after Tea. (Alcohol is the real #1, but it is the waste by-product of yeast.) One 8 oz. cup per day will bring caffeine which is a stimulant and will increase your metabolism and help burn calories. If you must sweeten it, use fresh Stevia. Coffee may be in this list but it is NOT the best way to go. If you already drink it, you should cut down to no more than one 8 oz. cup in the morning to get the ball rolling.[108]

9. DANDELION (Taraxacum officinale) – Already featured in the list of Diuretics (including a Recommended Supplement,) a recent study showed that Dandelion root does have a positive effect in weight loss. It is also a powerful detoxifier for the liver and is highly recommended. Products abound from supplements to herbal teas to dried root powder sold in bulk which is the most cost effective way to buy it.[78]

10. GRAPEFRUIT (Citrus paradisi) – King of the weight-loss foods. Grapefruit contains Synephrine which has a similar action to Ephedrine, a fad plant (Ephedra) and phytonutrient in the 1980's since banned due to the terrible side effects of overindulgence. While Synephrine is not nearly as powerful, it does increase fat burning metabolism and will definitely help you shed weight. It was the cornerstone of my own Natural Whole Foods Diet and it is very effective. Eat them whole, raw and do not add sugar. Tree ripened fruits are better tasting than store bought ones which are picked too green and stay very bitter and sour.[36]

11. GRAPES (Vitis vinifera) – Grapes contain a lot of powerful compounds including Anthocyanidins, Condensed Tannins, Myricetin and Resveratrol. That last one has been shown in at least one study to reduce the accumulation and production of adipose cells. The power is in the grape skins and anthocyanidins are dark colored antioxidants of enormous health benefit, so stick to red and black grapes. DO NOT OVERINDULGE; THE HIGH AMOUNTS OF TANNINS IN GRAPES, THE JUICE AND RAISINS CAN OVER TIME CAUSE KIDNEY PROBLEMS.[50]

12. GUARANA (Paullinia cupana) – This tropical plant contains Guaranine, a stimulant similar to caffeine and is used in some weight loss products. Because it is a stimulant, overindulgence can only lead to trouble. Try to find pure seed powder supplements or use the bulk powder to prepare herbal tea.[109]

RECOMMENDED GUARANA SUPPLEMENT
===

MANUFACTURER: SWANSON VITAMINS
PRODUCT NAME: PREMIUM GUARANA CAPSULES
WEBSITE: www. swansonvitamins.com
PRODUCT PAGE: www.swansonvitamins.com/swanson-premium-guarana-500-mg-100-caps

DO NOT OVERINDULGE IN GUARANA. NOT FOR LONG-TERM DAILY USE.

13. LICORICE (Glycyrrhiza glabra) – No modern store-bought product called "Licorice" actually contains any of the original plant and they are all now flavored by Anise (which is also good for you, by the way.) Licorice fell out of favor long ago because it can have terrible effects on human health if too much is consumed day after day. Licorice root is a tremendous health tonic that does increase metabolism and overindulgence is obviously not recommended. "Deglycyrrhizinated" licorice is useless for the purpose at hand which depends on the Glycyrrhizin, the main active constituent of Licorice root. Use with caution and avoid it if you have weak kidneys or high blood pressure, Licorice is strong and it will aggravate these issues in a DANGEROUS way.[110]

RECOMMENDED LICORICE ROOT SUPPLEMENT
===

MANUFACTURER: SWANSON VITAMINS
PRODUCT NAME: PREMIUM LICORICE ROOT
WEBSITE: www. swansonvitamins.com
PRODUCT PAGE: www.swansonvitamins.com/swanson-premium-licorice-root-450-mg-100-caps

DO NOT USE THIS HERB DAILY. Only use Licorice now and then because it is very potent. So much so that this is why all store-bought licorice no longer contains any of the real licorice plant in it any more: it caused SERIOUS HEALTH ISSUES in people that consumed it daily. DO NOT OVERINDULGE IN LICORICE. NOT FOR LONG-TERM DAILY USE.

14. LIME (Citrus aurantifolia) – Lime has been shown in at least one study to promote weight loss. Squeeze a Lime into other herbal teas or make a refreshing limeade daily. Its action is likely due to Synephrine which is found in the highest concentrations in Pomelo (C. maxima) and Grapefruit (also in this list.)[111]

15. LOTUS (Nelumbo nucifera and Nymphaea nouchali) – These two aquatic plant species are both called "Lotus," and both possess weight loss properties. Most parts of the plant are edible and increase metabolism, stimulate the burning of fat, prevent the formation of new adipose cells and inhibit pancreatic lipase and intestinal a-Glucosidase which reduces the calories from fats and sugars that the digestive tract absorbs from the meal. Fresh Lotus (either one) is not easy to locate, but if you can find it, it is good for your health.[112]

16. MUSHROOMS (Various species) – All edible mushrooms including: Agaricus blazei, Button or Portabella (Agaricus bisporus) Chaga (Inonotus obliquus) Enoki (Flammulina veluptis) Maitake (Grifola frondosa) Oyster (Pleurotus ostreatus) Reishi (Ganoderma lucidum) Shiitake (Lentinula edodes) Turkey Tail (Trametes versicolor) etc, contain a class of polysaccharides (complex sugar molecules) known as Beta-Glucans. Aside from numerous studies demonstrating their potent health benefits as immunostimulants and cancer fighters, they also assist with energy metabolism and may indeed help with weight loss. Even if they don't, the immune system benefits and their ability to actively combat some forms of cancer and their low calories make them ideal foods for everyone. Button (plain white) or Portabella are the same species and are readily available year round in most well stocked grocery stores. They are very low calorie and should be eaten raw in salad to prevent the heat of cooking from damaging the valuable beta-Glucans. (This is true of all edible mushrooms, by the way.)[115]

RECOMMENDED MAITAKE MUSHROOM SUPPLEMENT
==

MANUFACTURER: VITACOST
PRODUCT NAME: MAITAKE MUSHROOM EXTRACT
VENDOR WEBSITE: www.vitacost.com
PRODUCT PAGE: www.vitacost.com/vitacost-root2-maitake-mushroom-extract-standardized

Vitacost makes their own products and offers hundreds of other manufacturers' products for sale. They do not add chemicals or junk fillers.

17. NUT GRASS (Cyperus rotundus) – Oddly, you are much more likely to find this in a vacant lot than for sale in any form because it is considered the #1 most invasive weed on planet Earth and it is found everywhere. The rhizomes can be made into herbal tea that is apparently effective in reducing body fat due to the stimulation of fat burning metabolic processes.[116]

18. TANGERINE (Citrus tangerina) - This is the third Citrus fruit in the list and it should be clear that ALL of them are outstanding for good health, not just because of the Vitamin C, but for their many unique phytonutrients as well. Tangerines contain another unique compound called Nobelitin which is similar in activity to the Synephrine in Grapefruit, it stimulates fat metabolism and blocks the accumulation of fat in adipose cells. That's good news since store-bought Tangerines taste much better than store-bought grapefruit. Mandarins may also have this property.[208]

19. TEA (Camellia sinensis) – From a global perspective, Tea is likely the most abused consumable plant on Earth. The good news is that it is a stimulant, loaded with antioxidants, and it is also a diuretic and it is suspected of stimulating the burning of fat as well. Overindulgence is a very bad idea because tea is dark due to the Tannin content and too much Tannin will lead to kidney troubles that can get very serious. ONE 8 oz. cup per day should be the maximum. Green tea (made from fresh green leaves) does have a lower Tannin content and is generally safer, but the tannins are in there and OVERINDULGENCE IS NOT RECOMMENDED.[117]

CONCLUSION

Several plants in this list are readily available most of the year at your local well stocked grocery store and should be incorporated into your Natural Whole Foods Diet on a daily basis. Since Grapefruits and Tangerines are far more readily available than Pomelos and contain high concentrations of Synephrine in the case of Grapefruit and Nobelitin in the case of Tangerines which are well documented and scientifically verified stimulants of fat burning metabolism you must add these fruits to your diet. The more the better; I ate at least three Grapefruits a day while on my own weight loss diet and they were the nasty bitter and sour store bought ones. One 8 oz, cup of either coffee or tea is acceptable as are all edibles in this list especially the edible mushrooms. There are plenty of supplement products based on these mushrooms and many are fractions (partial extracts) and these are of dubious concentration and effect so try to find 100% pure dried powders or extracts. Fresh, raw, plain white Button or Portabella mushrooms in your salad are very low calorie and just too good for your health to pass up.

The term "Adaptogen" is relatively new and used to describe those medicinal herbs that in the past were usually lumped into the broad category called "Tonics." Like all holistic herbs, most of these plants have their own unique spread of active phytonutrients and some are stronger than others. Some will be very effective for one person and seemingly have no effect for another. It is entirely because of this behavior that many people become discouraged by the results they get with medicinal herbs and either give up or worse; they try to megadose on the plant to see if they can feel some slight effect. And more often than not, the person either has a bad reaction to the herb or abandons medicinal plants accusing them of being ineffective and nothing but hype.

Many holistic plants, both edible and medicinal can be used to make teas or can be taken in supplement form and are often so gentle that you won't feel anything overt, but that does not mean that they are not working and the adaptogens definitely fall into this category as opposed to the stimulants, for example, that often do have noticeable effects. The best bet is to take them in moderation for a while and trust them to do their job. Also, many adaptogens are actually quite strong and should not be used daily for long periods. These are intended for convalescence and recovery, like Ginseng, one of the least understood holistic herbs because of this property.

Many adaptogens are also immunostimulants. They are not recommended for those suffering from autoimmune disorders like LUPUS, or chronic infections like Hepatitis, HIV, or even cold/flu. If you have any of these maladies ASK YOUR DOCTOR BEFORE TAKING ANY IMMUNE STIMULANT.

THE ADAPTOGENS

1. ASHWAGANDHA (Withania somnifera) – The root of this plant has become very popular of late for its alleged effects in improving male sex drive which might be true. It is considered to be a non-specific health tonic with a milder action than Ginseng and is considered superior for infirmed and debilitated patients. Ashwagandha does promote deep restful sleep (hence the scientific name "somnifera" which means "makes you sleep") and is recommended for use at night.[75]

RECOMMENDED ASHWAGANDHA SUPPLEMENT
==

MANUFACTURER: SWANSON VITAMINS
PRODUCT NAME: PREMIUM ASHWAGANDHA
WEBSITE: www. swansonvitamins.com
PRODUCT PAGE: www.swansonvitamins.com/swanson-premium-ashwagandha-450-mg-100-caps

Although milder than Ginseng, LONG TERM USAGE OF THIS HERB IS NOT RECOMMENDED. Use as directed through one bottle. This should help you make a better transition to a low calorie Natural Whole Foods Diet.

2. ASTRAGALUS (Astragalus membranaceus) – This holistic herb has garnered a reputation in the past few decades as an effective adaptogen to fight chronic fatigue and as a potent immunostimulant. Astragalus has been shown to increase the production of Interferon which means that it can help fight viral infections especially respiratory afflictions. Astragalus has also been shown to be an effective heart tonic.[142]

RECOMMENDED ASTRAGALUS SUPPLEMENT
==

MANUFACTURER: SWANSON VITAMINS
PRODUCT NAME: PREMIUM ASTRAGALUS ROOT
WEBSITE: www. swansonvitamins.com
PRODUCT PAGE: www.swansonvitamins.com/swanson-premium-astragalus-root-470-mg-100-caps

This herb, like many adaptogens is an immunostimulant. As such it is NOT RECOMMENDED for those suffering from AUTOIMMUNE DISORDERS like some forms of ARTHRITIS or LUPUS, or viral INFECTIONS like HEPATITIS, HIV, or even COLD/FLU.

3. CELERY (Apium graviolens) – Celery, aside from being an excellent low calorie food, is also loaded with phytoestrogens and can help with various women's health issues, but it has also been shown in at least one study to also be an effective adaptogen in relieving the effects of physical stress and increasing endurance. Celery already makes the grade as an effective Diuretic and Net Negative Calorie Food, and is widely available year-round making it a true Top Recommended Superfood. Celery should be the cornerstone snack food for anyone trying to lose weight.[81]

4. CUT-LEAVED PANAX (Polyscias fruticosa) – The whole plant is edible and has a strong spicy flavor similar to celery or parsley and is both an immunostimulant and adaptogen. The problem is its lack of availability fresh or as supplements.[206]

5. DONG QUAI (Angelica sinensis) – Chinese Angelica is the second most revered holistic herb in Traditional Chinese Medicine after Ginseng. Like Angelica (A. archangelica) it has high amounts of phytoestrogens that can resolve many women's health issues. However, it is not just for women. The herbal tea decoction of the root is a strong diuretic and antibacterial. It is also a blood tonic, improves circulation, offers pain relief, acts as a tranquilizer, and protects the liver. It enhances the immune system by increasing production of white blood cells as well which might be the key to its recognized anticancer power. Dong Quai might fit into the category of general health tonic because it does have so many different health benefits, but its name means "Proper order" and it is used in many Traditional Chinese Medicine formulas for its capacity to restore a person to proper order likely by promoting hormonal balance and this is the true definition of an adaptogen.[146]

RECOMMENDED DONG QUAI SUPPLEMENT

MANUFACTURER: SWANSON VITAMINS
PRODUCT NAME: PREMIUM DONG QUAI ROOT
WEBSITE: www. swansonvitamins.com
PRODUCT PAGE: www.swansonvitamins.com/swanson-premium-dong-quai-root-530-mg-100-caps

This is an immunostimulant. IF YOU HAVE AN AUTOIMMUNE DISORDER OR A CHRONIC INFECTION, ASK YOUR DOCTOR BEFORE USING DONG QUAI.

6. ELECTRIC DAISY (Spilanthes acmella) – Extracts of this plant have shown the capacity to regulate the immune system and protect brain cells suggesting that it is a general effect adaptogen. The plant is more popular as an unusual garden flower than as a holistic herb and supplements may be hard to find.[147]

7. ELEUTHERO (Eleutherococcus senticosus) – A.k.a. Siberian ginseng although it is not related, does have similar properties and is considered milder than true Asian Ginseng. Eleuthero root can energize a person suffering from chronic fatigue and helps restore and protect the adrenal glands. It also boosts the immune system, and improves concentration and focus. Its greatest strength as an adaptogen is its ability to normalize hormone levels even when the body is under stress and it is the #1 adaptogen for those who decide to "go on a diet" by severely restricting their caloric intake. When this happens, the body will have a significant reaction and begin producing Cortisol and undergo other chemical changes that cause the body to protect the fat stores rather than give them up including lowering the metabolic rate.[148]

RECOMMENDED ELEUTHERO SUPPLEMENT

MANUFACTURER: SWANSON VITAMINS
PRODUCT NAME: PREMIUM ELEUTHERO ROOT
WEBSITE: www. swansonvitamins.com
PRODUCT PAGE: www.swansonvitamins.com/swanson-premium-eleuthero-root-425-mg-120-caps

Eleuthero specifically prevents the chemical changes incurred by "Famine Shock" (severe reduction in caloric intake) which often results in weight GAIN in the early stages of a calorie restricted diet that can be discouraging. Eleuthero root, available in dietary supplements as well as bulk dried powder, is one of the best ways to avoid this issue and is key to making your diet effective.

8. FEVER BARK (Alstonia scholaris) – The bark of this small shrub has been known for centuries and has a wide range of medicinal properties. As you might expect it is used to treat fevers but that is only the beginning. Because Fever Bark has such a wide range of health benefits it is considered a strong adaptogen however, and is not recommended for long term use. Supplements are very hard to find and might not be available in the U.S.[96]

9. FO-TI (Polygonum multiflorum) – In Traditional Chinese Medicine Fo-Ti root (He Shou-wu) is believed to be an anti-aging herb. It revitalizes those suffering from chronic fatigue and it said to return color to gray hair (possibly the origin of the immortality myth behind it) and it definitely falls into the category of general health tonic and adaptogen. Unprocessed root tea can be very harsh and is not recommended.[149]

RECOMMENDED FO-TI SUPPLEMENT

==

MANUFACTURER: SWANSON VITAMINS
PRODUCT NAME: PREMIUM FO-TI ROOT
WEBSITE: www. swansonvitamins.com
PRODUCT PAGE: www.swansonvitamins.com/swanson-premium-fo-ti-500-mg-60-caps

FO-TI IS NOT FOR DAILY USE, MODERATION IS ADVISED. FO-TI ROOT IS NOT RECOMMENDED FOR LONG-TERM USE.

10. GINGER (Zinziber officinale) – Ginger is one of the Big 3 best known medicinal herbs along with Aloe vera and Eucalyptus and has a long list of medicinal properties. For this alone it is considered a potent and safe adaptogen. Ginger helps prevent internal blood clotting, lowers blood pressure, improves circulation, lowers cholesterol, aids digestion by improving cell membrane permeability (helps the intestinal lining cells absorb nutrients) and helps to speed more active compounds from the rest of the meal into the blood stream – and that's just for starters! It is a known powerful antimicrobial as well. Cook with it daily and make herbal tea for general wellness.[150]

11. GINSENG (Panax ginseng) – Also called Asian Ginseng, to distinguish it from American Ginseng (P. quinquefolia,) this is probably one of the least understood holistic herbs. It is a powerful restorative tonic and a potent immunostimulant ideal for those who are convalescing due to chronic illness, fatigue, or debilitation. DO NOT USE Ginseng if you suffer from high blood pressure or are taking high blood pressure or cholesterol medication.[151]

RECOMMENDED GINSENG SUPPLEMENT

==

MANUFACTURER: SWANSON VITAMINS
PRODUCT NAME: PREMIUM GINSENG ROOT
WEBSITE: www. swansonvitamins.com
PRODUCT PAGE: www.swansonvitamins.com/swanson-premium-korean-ginseng-500-mg-100-caps

MODERATION IS ADVISED because Ginseng is VERY STRONG MEDICINE and NOT RECOMMENDED FOR LONG-TERM USE.

12. HOG PLUM (Spondias pinnata) – Although this fruit is not considered to have the nutritional value of most others, one study did demonstrate that it does have significant antioxidant content and a measurable reduction of physical stress levels and it helped mitigate the effects of a chemical immunosuppressant making it a notable adaptogen. These fruits might be available on rare occasion at a farmer's market. Hog Plum based products and supplements may not exist.[152]

13. HOG WEED (Boerhavia diffusa) – Aside from having edible leaves, one study showed that extracts of this plant were able to increase endurance. Many plants go by this name, so verification of the species is important. This plant is admittedly difficult to find for sale in any form.[103]

14. HOLY BASIL (Ocimum sanctum) – Used for thousands of years in the Ayurvedic traditions of India, Holy Basil, a.k.a. Tulsi, is a close relative to culinary Basil and is a powerful adaptogen with many health benefits. Studies have shown that it is a verified and powerful neuroprotective that can help prevent degenerative brain diseases like Alzheimer's.[153]

RECOMMENDED HOLY BASIL SUPPLEMENT
==

MANUFACTURER: SWANSON VITAMINS
PRODUCT NAME: SUPERIOR HERBS HOLY BASIL
WEBSITE: www. swansonvitamins.com
PRODUCT PAGE: www.swansonvitamins.com/swanson-superior-herbs-holy-basil-extract-tulsi-400-mg-60-caps

Holy Basil is essentially a spice and despite its strength it is relatively safe to use but, MODERATION IS ADVISED.

15. HYSSOP (Hyssopus officinalis) – Hyssop has a historical reputation as an antimicrobial and is used for cold/flu, cough, and other respiratory ailments. Because it is highly volatile, making the tea should be done in a closed vessel to help preserve the active compounds. Hyssop is not as well known as a general tonic or adaptogen as most of the others in this list and it does contain ketones that can become toxic in excess so it is not for long-term or heavy daily usage.[105]

RECOMMENDED HYSSOP SUPPLEMENT
==

MANUFACTURER: SWANSON VITAMINS
PRODUCT NAME: PREMIUM HYSSOP
WEBSITE: www. swansonvitamins.com
PRODUCT PAGE: www.swansonvitamins.com/swanson-premium-hyssop-450-mg-100-caps

Because of the potentially toxic ketones, and the fact that its main use is for respiratory infections, HYSSOP SHOULD BE USED VERY SPARINGLY. HYSSOP IS NOT FOR LONG-TERM USE.

16. JIAOGULAN (Gynostemma pentaphyllum): This is another well known Traditional Chinese Medicine herb with a legendary reputation as a health and longevity tonic. It is a very effective immunostimulant, adaptogen, vasodilator, and supplements abound. Studies have also shown its ability to normalize blood pressure, and help in weight-loss programs. Called Amachazuru in

Japan which means "Sweet tea vine," the leaves of this close relative to cucumber are used to make healthy herbal tea. [106]

TOP RECOMMENDED JIAOGULAN SUPPLEMENT
==

MANUFACTURER: Paradise Herbs
PRODUCT NAME: Jiaogulan 60 Veg Capsules
VENDOR WEBSITE: www.vitacost.com

17. MACA ROOT (Lepidium peruvianum) – Maca is an edible root tuber or rhizome of a tropical vine related to radishes and is a staple food in some South American regions. In those regions it also has a reputation of being an energy tonic and studies have shown that it may be a significant immunostimulant. Maca root is also loaded with phytoestrogens and can help with women's health issues and like all such plants it should not be used by nursing or pregnant mothers. Supplements are getting expensive because the plant is becoming endangered and only grows in the South American mountains above 12,000 feet and there are no efforts by the local communities to set up large scale production and they also do not want it exported live for cultivation elsewhere.[154]

RECOMMENDED MACA ROOT SUPPLEMENT
==

MANUFACTURER: SWANSON VITAMINS
PRODUCT NAME: PREMIUM HYSSOP
WEBSITE: www. swansonvitamins.com
PRODUCT PAGE: www.swansonvitamins.com/swanson-premium-maca-500-mg-100-caps

Maca is edible and considered relatively safe, but it is likely to go up in price because the plant is not being properly preserved or cultivated in its native range.

18. MAITAKE MUSHROOM (Grifola frondosa) – All edible mushrooms contain forms of polysaccharides (complex sugars) known as Beta-Glucans. Numerous laboratory tests and clinical trials have confirmed that these unusual molecules built from simple sugars act as powerful immunostimulants and combat the formation of tumors and can combat established tumors as well. Maitake in particular also protects the liver, lowers blood pressure, and lowers blood sugar levels and it is believed that it may also help with weight loss. Despite being powerful medicine, Maitake is edible and relatively safe compared to most other adaptogens, immunostimulants and anticancer holistic herbs and comes highly recommended. There are plenty of supplements and herbal teas to choose from and these are a way to get in on this mushroom's enormous health benefits because most gourmet mushrooms have gone way up in price now that science backs their health promoting reputations. By the way, both Button (plain white) and Portabella mushrooms are the same species (Agaricus bisporus) and they also contain Beta-Glucans. They are best raw in salad because cooking could damage the desired beta-Glucans.[115]

19. OATS (Avena sativa) – One of the few true plants that also contains Beta-Glucans and thus brings the same health benefits as the edible mushrooms, Oats, specifically "Old-fashioned" oatmeal, should be the only breakfast cereal on the menu during your process of conversion to a Natural Whole Foods Diet while replacing poor quality packaged, processed foods with natural high quality "Functional" foods (high in nutritional and/or medicinal value.) Oatmeal also brings some vitamins and minerals and while it does have more calories than the NNC foods, it is worth it and because of the high Dietary Fiber content; it is very filling.[68]

20. PEPPERMINT (Mentha piperita) – Mint has many health benefits, so much so that it is considered an adaptogen. It is antibacterial, antifungal, antiviral, and that is just the beginning. But this does not mean toothpaste, candy or green packaged cigarettes all of which are flavored by a single manufactured chemical (Menthol.) Leaves of the REAL peppermint plant either in the essential oil, extracts, or used to make herbal tea contain hundreds of compounds and it is this group that brings all of the health benefits. Live plants and 100% pure natural products abound and are highly recommended. However, overindulgence is a bad idea; mint is a vasoconstrictor (causes blood vessels and capillaries to constrict raising blood pressure) and a rubifacient (contact irritant.)[155]

RECOMMENDED PEPPERMINT SUPPLEMENT
==

MANUFACTURER: SWANSON VITAMINS
PRODUCT NAME: FULL SPECTRUM PEPPERMINT
WEBSITE: www. swansonvitamins.com
PRODUCT PAGE: www.swansonvitamins.com/swanson-premium-full-spectrum-peppermint-leaf-400-mg-120-caps

Fresh mint leaf tea is far superior because many of its active compounds are volatile and evaporate during the making of any natural mint product.

21. RHODIOLA (Rhodiola rosea) – Like many adaptogens, Rhodiola makes the list because it is both a stimulant and an immunostimulant. Recent studies have shown that it is effective in improving brain function and is helps in cases of mild to moderate depression. Being somewhat potent, moderation is advised.[156]

TOP RECOMMENDED RHODIOLA SUPPLEMENT
==

MANUFACTURER: NOW FOODS
PRODUCT NAME: RHODIOLA 500mg
WEBSITE: www.nowfoods.com
PRODUCT PAGE: www.nowfoods.com/supplements/Rhodiola-500-mg-veg-capsules

If you have an AUTOIMMUNE DISORDER or an INFECTION ASK YOUR DOCTOR BEFORE USING RHODIOLA. Because it is a stimulant, RHODIOLA IS NOT FOR LONG-TERM DAILY USE.

22. SCHISANDRA (Schisandra chinensis) – This is a climbing vine that produces edible berries that have a long revered history in Traditional Chinese Medicine. The Chinese call it "Wu wei zi" meaning the Five Tastes because it is sour, bitter, sweet, warm and salty. Schisandra berry enhances immune function, relieves chronic fatigue, improves endurance, and is a lung tonic and can improve breathing. Schisandra has been shown in studies to help regenerate liver tissue and has been used in China to treat a form of hepatitis. It is loaded with anthocyanidins (powerful antioxidants) and supports eye health. Sundry products are available and highly recommended, but try to get as close to pure and unadulterated as you can (i.e. 100% pure juice or extracts.)[157]

TOP RECOMMENDED SCHISANDRA PRODUCTS
==
MANUFACTURER: NATURE'S WAY
PRODUCT NAME: SCHISANDRA FRUIT 580mg
VENDOR WEBSITE: www. swansonvitamins.com
PRODUCT PAGE: www.swansonvitamins.com/natures-way-schizandra-fruit-580-mg-100-caps
You can buy this product directly from Nature's Way at their own website: www.naturesway.com.
==
MANUFACTURER: MOUNTAIN ROSE HERBS
PRODUCT NAME: SCHISANDRA BERRY POWDER
VENDOR WEBSITE: www. mountainroseherbs.com
PRODUCT PAGE: www.mountainroseherbs.com/products/schisandra-berry-powder/profile
This product is expensive but it is pure and probably the highest quality you will find. Most others will be mixed with other cheaper fruits and are not worth the expense.

23. SUMA ROOT (Pfaffia paniculata) – A.k.a. Brazilian Ginseng, this is a true adaptogen although it is not related to true Ginseng, it is actually related to Amaranth. Suma root helps the body deal with stress (like significant changes to diet,) increases energy levels and resistance to disease. From this we assume that it helps regulate hormone levels, increases metabolism and is an immunostimulant. Limited studies in the 1970's showed some anticancer properties as well although there has been little work done on this particular plant since then. Powdered Suma root has a spicy Vanilla flavor and makes a delicious herbal tea. Products are available and bulk dried root is probably the best way to go and it comes highly recommended but since there has been very little study of the plant, overindulgence is not recommended.[158]

RECOMMENDED SUMA ROOT SUPPLEMENT
==
MANUFACTURER: SWANSON VITAMINS
PRODUCT NAME: FULL SPECTRUM SUMA ROOT
WEBSITE: www. swansonvitamins.com

PRODUCT PAGE: www.swansonvitamins.com/swanson-premium-full-spectrum-suma-root-400-mg-60-caps
Since little recent study has been done with Suma Root, its safety is unknown. OVERINDULGENCE IS NOT RECOMMENDED.

CONCLUSION

For those who have suffered the frustration of going on a diet only to gain weight, the adaptogens are definitely the answer to this frustrating problem. Science has confirmed that sudden severe reductions in calories causes the body to go into "Famine shock" and produce Cortisol and other hormones intended to reduce metabolic rate to conserve energy and to protect the fat cells from giving up their stores. While this might be a useful evolutionary development, it is not very useful for a person who wants to lose those extra unwanted pounds.

Aside from the edible plants in this list, notably Celery, Ginger, Maitake (or store-bought Button or Portabella) Mushrooms, Oats, Peppermint leaves, and Schisandra Berry, the most effective adaptogens for weight loss are in order of priority: Eleuthero, Jiaogulan, Dong Quai, Suma Root, and Rhodiola. But the others are quite useful as well bringing a wide range of additional health benefits including protection of the brain cells, liver protection, immune boosters, etc. And as with all natural plants some will work for one person while having little effect for another. Because of this, it is often necessary to try various plants until you find the ones that are the most effective for YOU. Just don't try them all at once! It might work, but you won't know which ones are effective.

Some of these work by inhibiting the appetite, while others work by inhibiting the formation of adipose (fat storage) cells and may even work to reduce their numbers (encourage the body to burn the fat.)

1. ACEROLA (Malpighia punicifolia) – Acerola berry, a.k.a. West Indian Cherry, has the highest concentration of Vitamin C found in any natural food. Just one small berry has about 100% of the RDA amount. Acerola products abound but are often adulterated with other fruits and should not be so expensive since there may be very little Acerola in them. Pure Acerola juice has been shown to help reduce inflammation and ameliorate the effects of a high fat diet.[118]

RECOMMENDED ACEROLA PRODUCT

==

MANUFACTURER: Microingredients
PRODUCT NAME: ORGANIC ACEROLA POWDER
VENDOR'S HOST WEBSITE: www.amazon.com
PRODUCT PAGE: www.amazon.com/Organic-Cherries-Powerful-Non-Irradiated-Friendly/dp/B06XC72G8G

This product is dried fruit powder and can be used to make the straight drink with water, or can be added to other drinks to get in on the health benefits of Acerola. The seller is only being hosted at Amazon (like eBay) and their trustworthiness is unknown.

2. AVOCADO (Persea Americana) – Some studies have shown that Avocado has the ability to lower cholesterol and blood sugar levels. It does bring a lot of calories, but in the form of complex sugars and Monounsaturated Fats. Research has shown that some of these unusual fats assist in the absorption of Carotenes like beta-Carotene in Carrots and Lycopene in Tomatoes. They also actually promote the conversion of beta-Carotene (and others) into Vitamin A. Finally, Avocado's unusual sugars and fats increase satiety. Eating Avocado causes you to feel full faster and retain that feeling longer which is a boon for folks trying to lose weight. Add a slice to the lunch salad along with shredded Carrot and sliced Tomato to take full advantage of its ability to help absorb their powerful antioxidant Carotenes.[209]

3. CANTALOUPE (Cucumis melo) – This wonderful relative of the Cucumber has shown in studies the ability to lower total cholesterol, lower LDL (the "bad") cholesterol, lower triglycerides, as well as the ability to interfere with lipid metabolism and the formation of new adipose cells. Cantaloupe is also loaded with Carotenoid antioxidants and should definitely be on the menu.[210]

4. CHIA SEED (Salvia hispanica) – Numerous studies have shown that Chia seed reduces cholesterol and blood glucose levels. It has also been shown to improve satiety and is the best source of the plant Omega-3 Fatty Acid – alpha-Linoleic Acid and also a great source of Dietary Fiber. When included in any meal studies have shown that it reduced the Glycemic Index of the entire meal apparently by slowing the absorption of simple sugars in the digestive tract. Add some ground Chia seed to the morning Oatmeal as an excellent way to include it in your daily diet.[59]

5. CHICKWEED (Stellaria media) – Chickweed leaves are edible raw in salads and Chickweed is a well known anti-inflammatory that can be made into poultices or herbal tea which is also known for its appetite suppression property.[119]

RECOMMENDED CHICKWEED SUPPLEMENT
=======================================

MANUFACTURER: SWANSON VITAMINS
PRODUCT NAME: PREMIUM CHICKWEED CAPSULES
WEBSITE: www. swansonvitamins.com
PRODUCT PAGE: www.swansonvitamins.com/swanson-premium-chickweed-450-mg-180-caps

6. COLEUS (Coleus forskohlii) – Coleus is powerful medicine, so much so that trying to use this close relative to Basil fresh from the garden is not recommended because getting the dose correct is nearly impossible. Supplements abound and it is most famous for its proven powerful immunostimulant effect however, it also acts as an appetite suppressant, helps properly absorb all nutrients, aids the breakdown of fats, and lowers cholesterol.[88]

TOP RECOMMENDED COLEUS SUPPLEMENT
=======================================

MANUFACTURER: VITACOST
PRODUCT NAME: Coleus Forskohlii Extract
WEBSITE: www.vitacost.com

Coleus is powerful medicine and a confirmed immunostimulant. If you suffer from any chronic infection including Hepatitis, HIV, or are currently suffering from cold/flu, etc, ASK YOUR DOCTOR BEFORE TAKING COLEUS or any other IMMUNE STIMULANT.

7. DARK CHOCOLATE (Theobroma cacao) – This is certainly good news for anyone on a diet! Dark Chocolate is a Superfood. Four ounces brings 100% RDA amounts of BOTH Iron and Magnesium, two minerals that are hard to get in those amounts from natural whole foods on a daily basis. However, four ounces also brings 180% RDA of COPPER and that is TOO MUCH. It is also loaded with Tannins which can put a strain on the kidneys and four ounces bring 560 calories. However, ONE ounce per day will bring the stimulant Theobromine which is similar to caffeine without the negative affect of disrupting sleep. Real chocolate (we are NOT talking about candy here) also brings Phenylethylamine (PEA) and Anandamide. PEA stimulates the release of Dopamine which is what makes a person happy when they eat chocolate and Anandamide is a neurotransmitter that enhances and prolongs this effect. Researchers believe that chocolate, despite being so heavy with fat calories has a "Net Negative" impact on caloric intake; it enhances mood, happiness and satisfaction allowing a person to go for longer periods of time without craving MORE "comfort food" and actually results in less total calories consumed throughout the course of the day: just be sure to keep it at no more than 2 ounces per day. Pure 100% Cacao as Unsweetened Baker's Chocolate Bars is the real thing; just read the ingredients label which should consist of ONE item: Chocolate. Sweeten it with a touch of 100% Pure Raw Bee Honey which is also very good for you.[57]

8. DATES (Phoenix dactylifera) – Date palms have one of the slowest maturity rates of all flowering plants. The palms take up to eighty years to mature and bear fruit and the vast majority of the Earth's supply comes from Sri Lanka. Dates have been shown to significantly lower cholesterol levels and have a positive effect on weight loss although the mechanism of this action is still unknown. Despite being so sweet they have an average Glycemic Index of 42±4 which is very good for such a sweet sun-dried fruit.[211]

9. DRAGON FRUIT (Hylocereus undatus) – If you have never had a Dragon Fruit, you should definitely try one. As strange as they look (they are aptly named, and look like a Dragon egg) the plant is even more bizarre: it is a cactus, and a VINE. They form a tangle of long thin cactus segments that will climb a strong trellis. Dragon fruit contains compounds that lower blood sugar, reduce insulin resistance and most importantly to this discussion: promote fat burning metabolism.[212]

10. FENNEL (Foeniculum vulgare) – Fennel has a long historical reputation as a weight loss herb mainly due to its ability to curb the appetite. You can make Fennel seed tea from the ground or whole seed spice found in most well stocked grocery stores and drink it 15 minutes before a meal and it reportedly will curb your appetite. It is also believed to help properly absorb and convert fats into smaller molecules that can be used for energy immediately rather than leaving them in forms that the body would be more likely to store instead.[121]

11. GAMBOGE (Garcinia gambogia) – This is another fad plant that has risen in fame in the last two decades and rightfully so. It also goes by many different names including Garcinia, Camboga, and Cambogia. Its power comes from the Hydroxycitric Acid which has been shown in studies to curb the appetite and help prevent the formation of fat within the body. HCA in supplements is bound to calcium (Calcium Hydroxycitrate) and is not easily absorbed meaning supplements based on this form will have limited effect. Try to find fresh juice or natural extracts of the fruit.[122]

RECOMMENDED GAMBOGE SUPPLEMENT
==

MANUFACTURER: SWANSON VITAMINS
PRODUCT NAME: PREMIUM GARCINIA CAMBOGIA
WEBSITE: www. swansonvitamins.com
PRODUCT PAGE: www.swansonvitamins.com/swanson-premium-garcinia-cambogia-5-1-extract-80-mg-60-caps

12. GARDENIA (Gardenia jasminoides) – One of the more popular garden shrubs, Gardenia flowers as well as the fruits and roots have been well studied for their many interesting and powerful health benefits attributed to several unique compounds including Crocin, Crocetin, Genipin and Geniposide. Studies suggest that it has a strong positive action for the Pancreas (quite rare) as well as the Liver. Gardenia flower tea can reduce blood cholesterol and has a strong anti-diabetic action. It is also a strong antioxidant, anti-inflammatory, gastroprotective, and has shown anti-depressive effects as well as the potential to protect brain cells from the kind of oxidative damage that leads to Alzheimer's disease. A study also noted that it is a strong Pancreatic Lipase inhibitor and can quickly reverse obesity. Gardenia is STRONG medicine, add ONE fresh flower to your regular dark tea every other day to see if it works for you.[213]

13. GARLIC (Allium sativa) – The health benefits of Garlic are sundry and impressive. Its main active ingredient is Allicin which gives it that unmistakable aroma and flavor, but it is loaded with other Glucosinolates (Sulfur-containing organic compounds) including Organosulfur which is a ring of eight sulfur atoms. This is far safer than plain elemental sulfur which can turn extremely TOXIC in the stomach. Garlic lowers blood pressure and reduces the risk of internal blood clotting by inhibiting the platelets from sticking to each other or blood vessel surfaces; it also reduces LDL's (the bad forms of cholesterol) in the blood and helps with the digestion of fats which is key to this discussion. Any food that assists in the breakdown of fats means that fewer fat molecules will make it through to the liver which reduces the numbers of them that will end up in the adipose cells for storage.[99]

14. GURMAR (Gymnema sylvestre) – Used for thousands of years in the Ayurvedic medicinal tradition of India, Gurmar, rarely sold by this original Ayurvedic name, has many health benefits including helping to curb the desire for sugar and sweets. It also helps to control blood sugar levels and is excellent for prevention and control of Type II diabetes. Gurmar also helps to normalize blood cholesterol levels.[123]

RECOMMENDED GURMAR SUPPLEMENT
==

MANUFACTURER: SWANSON VITAMINS
PRODUCT NAME: PREMIUM GYMNEMA SYLVESTRE
WEBSITE: www. swansonvitamins.com
PRODUCT PAGE: www.swansonvitamins.com/swanson-premium-gymnema-sylvestre-leaf-400-mg-100-caps

15. HEAVENLY ELIXIR (Tinospora crispa) – Extracts of this plant's leaves and stems have one of the longest lists of medicinal properties of all holistic plants, hence the name. Among many other health benefits at least one study has shown that it helps reduce body fat. While it is a potent medicine, long term usage is not recommended. Supplements are admittedly difficult to find and may not be available in the U.S.[124]

16. HIBISCUS (Hibiscus sabdariffa) – Hibiscus tea is made from the flowers, but go easy on it, because it is powerful medicine. Add two ounces of fresh flowers in one pint of hot water and let it steep for about ten minutes then drink no more than one 8 oz. cup and no more than twice a week. Hibiscus will definitely lower blood pressure. Hibiscus like Gamboge has Hydroxycitric Acid in it which suppresses the appetite and inhibits the formation of fat in the adipose cells.[102]

RECOMMENDED HIBISCUS SUPPLEMENT
==

MANUFACTURER: SWANSON VITAMINS
PRODUCT NAME: PREMIUM HIBISCUS FLOWER
WEBSITE: www. swansonvitamins.com
PRODUCT PAGE: www.swansonvitamins.com/swanson-premium-full-spectrum-hibiscus-flower-400-mg-60-caps

TOP RECOMMENDED HIBISCUS TEA
==

MANUFACTURER: NOW FOODS
PRODUCT NAME: ORGANICALLY HIP HIBISCUS TEA
WEBSITE: www.nowfoods.com
PRODUCT PAGE: www.nowfoods.com/natural-foods/
organically-hip-hibiscus-tea

HIBISCUS IS STRONG MEDICINE, MODERATION IS ADVISED. DO NOT USE HIBISCUS IF YOU ARE TAKING HIGH BLOOD PRESSURE OR CHOLESTEROL MEDICATION OR BLOOD THINNERS. ASK YOUR DOCTOR BEFORE USING HIBISCUS.

17. HOODIA (Hoodia gordonii) – The main problem with this plant is that it comes from southern Africa where it is endangered from over-harvesting and the locals do not want the plant to be exported for cultivation. All of this means that the products are expensive and only bound to go up in price. Hoodia is a succulent that looks very much like a cactus, and fresh as well as powdered products are likely safe and it is a potent appetite suppressant. Most western products are fractions of the extract and are not as effective despite the hype.[125]

RECOMMENDED HOODIA SUPPLEMENT
==

MANUFACTURER: SWANSON VITAMINS
PRODUCT NAME: FULL SPECTRUM HOODIA GORDONII
WEBSITE: www. swansonvitamins.com
PRODUCT PAGE: www.swansonvitamins.com/swanson-premium-full-spectrum-hoodia-gordonii-400-mg-180-caps

18. JABOTICABA (Myrciaria cauliflora) – This rare fruit from Brazil is starting to gain popularity. It is actually a relative of the common Cherry Hedge (Surinam Cherry: Eugenia multiflora) although it grows much more slowly. The fruits resemble large black grapes and are said to taste like grapes as well. Preliminary tests have shown that the Jaboticaba fruit does help reduce body fat although the mechanism is still unknown. Jaboticaba fruit, if you can find it, has a very high antioxidant content as well.[51]

19. JEW'S MALLOW (Corchorus olitorius) – This is a popular vegetable in the Philippines, young shoots and leaves are edible when cooked and it has been shown in at least one study to have a significant effect in reducing body fat. One source indicates that supplements are available but they may be difficult to find.[126]

20. JOB'S TEARS (Coix lachryma) – Also known as Asian barley, supplements are very hard to find, but the flour is available. Extracts have shown the ability to inhibit neuroendocrine activity which leads to reduced body fat. If you like to bake, using Job's Tears flour to make biscuits, flatbread, etc. would be an excellent substitute for plain bleached white wheat flour goods.[107]

21. JUJUBE (Ziziphus jujuba) – This is one of the best functional foods on Earth and one of the very best trees to grow at home if you have the land. Jujube trees have no known diseases, are flood tolerant, draught tolerant, heat tolerant (they are found in deserts) and they are also deciduous (can survive severe freezing winters.) They are covered in hard thin tiny thorns that are extremely sharp, but the fruit has shown effective weight loss properties and also lowers cholesterol.[127]

RECOMMENDED JUJUBE SUPPLEMENT
==

MANUFACTURER: SWANSON VITAMINS
PRODUCT NAME: FULL SPECTRUM JUJUBE FRUIT
WEBSITE: www.swansonvitamins.com
PRODUCT PAGE: www.swansonvitamins.com/swanson-premium-full-spectrum-jujube-fruit-675-mg-60-caps

The dried fruit is preferable and might be available at your local Chinese grocery store (there are none within 50 miles of where I live.) The trees are native to China where the dried fruit (which is said to taste like Dates) is highly prized.

22. JUNIPER (Juniperus chinensis) – Juniper berry, already in the preceding list of Diuretics, as well as stem and leaf extracts have been shown in at least one study to inhibit adipose cell formation. Be absolutely sure you have the correct species if you try to make your own tea with the dried berries. MODERATION IS ADVISED. DAILY OVERINDULGENCE CAN LEAD TO KIDNEY DAMAGE.[84]

23. KELP (various spp.) – All species of Kelp are oceanic Brown Algae that share two well known characteristics: they are high in Iodine, and extremely low calorie. Some species may contain Vitamin B12, but if they do, it is best to take B12 supplements that contain the B12 extracted from the Kelp rather than depend on the whole plant to deliver it. This is mainly because the plants are extremely variable in Iodine content with some of them holding over 2000% RDA amounts per ounce which is enough to cause an adverse reaction for some people. Kelp contains several unique phytonutrients (Algae are true plants, just very simple ones) that promote weight loss. Fucoxanthin reduces fat tissue. Alginates present in varying amounts depending on the species inhibit pancreatic enzymes that promote the absorption of fat. Kelp also has anti-inflammatory, anti-diabetic and anti-cancer compounds of enormous interest to medical science.[214]

RECOMMENDED KELP SUPPLEMENT
===

MANUFACTURER: NOW FOODS
PRODUCT NAME: ORGANIC KELP POWDER
WEBSITE: www.nowfoods.com
PRODUCT PAGE: www.nowfoods.com/supplements/kelp-powder-organic

24. LIMA BEANS (Phaseolus lunatis) – One of the most hated of all beans, Lima beans have TWO exceptional health beneficial qualities: 1) They inhibit the absorption of simple sugars in the intestine which in turn leads to fewer calories actually absorbed from the meal, and 2) They contain a substance that counters ACE (Angiotensin Converting Enzyme) which the body produces to cause the blood vessels to constrict. By relaxing the blood vessels the blood pressure is lowered reducing the strain on the heart making these one of the best of the antihypertensive functional foods on Earth. They have an added bonus because they are relatively low calorie and featured in the Net Negative Calorie Foods list as well. If you already take an ACE inhibiting high blood pressure medication, CHECK WITH YOUR DOCTOR before adding Lima Beans to your diet.[128]

25. MANGOSTEEN (Garcinia mangostana) – This close relative of the Gamboge is one of the rarest fruits on Earth. It has very finicky environmental requirements and is difficult to grow outside of its native range in the South American highlands. It might be an embellishment based on its rarity, but many people insist that it might be the best tasting fruit on Earth. In addition to its fame, it has also been shown in studies to inhibit the liver from generating Triglycerides and Cholesterol and it also inhibits alpha-amylase in the intestines which in turn reduces the amounts of sugars that are absorbed. If you can find the fruit it will be pricey, but it might be worth a try just to see if it is as good as they say.[215]

26. NEW ZEALAND SPINACH (Tetragonia tetragonioides) – An excellent edible leafy vegetable, New Zealand Spinach has been shown to reduce body fat and inhibit the growth and formation of adipose cells. New Zealand Spinach is a true Functional food and it has a long history of use in holism as a treatment for women's hormonal imbalance issues and at just 3.3 cal per oz, it is one of the best Net Negative Calorie foods and edible raw in salads or steamed or boiled is a superb side dish for dinner that brings the added bonus of proactively helping you to lose weight by inhibiting the formation of fat cells. It is not often found in grocery stores so you might have to grow your own.[129]

27. ONIONS (Allium cepa) – Although many people tend to avoid onions because of the bad breath they cause, that is a tragic mistake. Aside from being excellent low calorie foods they are high in sulfur compounds that the body desperately needs and they have been shown to inhibit Fatty Acid Synthase, a key enzyme in the growth and formation of adipose cells. Onions will definitely help you lose weight. You can add onions, minced garlic, chives and/or scallions to the lunch salad. Raw chopped onion bulbs generate a detrimental compound but it does dissipate after a few minutes. Cooked into soups and stews they are very safe and excellent for your health.[130]

28. OREGANO (Origanum vulgare) – Most people associate Oregano with Italian cuisine, but it has scientifically proven health benefits. The main constituents are Carvacrol, Rosmarinic Acid and Thymol. These three compounds, aside from being potent antimicrobial agents help improve circulation and have been shown to help prevent cancer, cardiovascular disease and stroke. Oregano has one of the highest ORAC scores of any edible item at the grocery store (175,296 dried) and also has significant anti-inflammatory and anti-diabetic properties as well. It is also a mild stimulant which is what puts it in this list, but even if it didn't have that property, its myriad and significant health promoting powers are too good to pass up.[216]

29. PEANUTS (Arachis hypogaea) – I would have never guessed that Peanuts could be good for LOSING weight. But there is a catch; the active compounds are in the shells, not the kernels. This means that good ol' Southern style Boiled Peanuts which keeps the shells is the only way to get in on their weight-loss properties. But you will have to cook them yourself because most traditional Boiled Peanuts are cooked in salt saturated brine which has far too much Sodium that will cause high blood pressure.[33]

30. PRICKLY PEAR (Opuntia ficus-indica) – Prickly Pear cactus is one of the true wonders of the plant kingdom. It provides many nutrients including Calcium, Magnesium, and eight of the nine essential amino acids. Quercitin, Kaempferol, and Isorhamnetin are powerful antioxidants found in the plant that have been shown to possess anticancer properties. The Betalains, Carotenoids, and Polyphenols are all potent compounds with numerous studies demonstrating various health benefits. The Pectin and water-soluble Dietary Fiber have been shown to help counteract Type II diabetes, promote weight loss and lower LDL cholesterol levels in the blood. Both the fruits and the pads are edible, nutritious and powerful, safe medicine.[131]

31. PSYLLIUM (Plantago psyllium) – This close relative of the Plantain herb featured in the diuretics list is prized for its seeds.

Psyllium seed and seed husks are very high in dietary fiber (water-soluble, or the "Good" kind) and are typically used by herbalists to treat either diarrhea or constipation. No manmade chemical can relieve EITHER problem and that tells you everything you need to know about the power and gentleness of Dietary Fiber. Add good natural dietary fiber to your diet because it blocks the absorption of cholesterol from the meal and thus lowers cholesterol and blood triglyceride levels and it helps condition the intestinal lining as well. Psyllium is available in most pharmacies and because it is so high in fiber you should take small amounts a couple times a day.[132]

32. ROOIBOS TEA (Aspalathus linearis) – After centuries of use, there have been no reported cases of toxicity concerning this plants dried leaves which turn a rich crimson and yield a sweet, fruity flavored tea that is invigorating due to a mild stimulant effect. Because it contains Tannins which can be harsh for the kidneys, moderation is advised.[207]

TOP RECOMMENDED ROOIBOS TEA PRODUCT
===

MANUFACTURER: Choice Organic Teas
PRODUCT NAME: Rooibos Red Bush Tea
WEBSITE: http://www.swansonvitamins.com/
PRODUCT PAGE: https://www.swansonvitamins.com/choice-organic-teas-rooibos-red-bush-tea-caffeine-free-16-bags-s

33. ROSEMARY (Rosmarinus officinalis) – Rosemary is another common spice that has enormous health benefits. It has been shown to have weight loss properties along with many other health benefits and is also included in the Diuretics list. Cook often with it and it can also be used to make herbal tea. The best way to make Rosemary tea would be as a decoction by boiling it for about 20 to 30 minutes. You can also add ONE DROP of the essential oil to any other tea but only if it is 100% pure and not mixed with other oils intended for external use only.[94]

34. SAFFLOWER OIL (Carthamus tinctorius) – Safflower Oil has one of the highest concentrations of Conjugated Linoleic Acid or CLA which is commonly added to weight loss supplements and studies have shown that as a supplement it does have a marked effect in weight loss. Store bought brands of the cooking oil are too refined and therefore depleted of this important essential nutrient that the body cannot make on its own, so try to find Extra Virgin oil or supplements of either the oil or the Conjugated Linoleic Acid usually just called CLA.[133]

TOP RECOMMENDED CLA SUPPLEMENT
===

MANUFACTURER: NOW FOODS
PRODUCT NAME: CLA (Conjugated Linoleic Acid) Softgels
WEBSITE: www.nowfoods.com
PRODUCT PAGE: www.nowfoods.com/supplements/
cla-conjugated-linoleic-acid-800-mg-softgels

35. SAGE (Salvia officinalis) – Sage has a long list of health benefits including the ability to inhibit the accumulation of fat in adipose cells. Sage also contains Perillyl Alcohol which is currently under investigation for its ability to fight certain forms of brain cancer. Sage is common and a Top Recommended Spice. Use often in cooking or as herbal tea.[134]

36. SMARTWEED (Persicaria hydropiper) – This plant and possibly Knotweed (P. barbatus) contain Isoquercitrin which has been shown to inhibit the production of new adipocytes which can help with weight loss and prevent the formation of cellulite. Both plants are unfortunately hard to find in supplement form.[135]

37. STAR FRUIT (Averrhoa carambola) – Studies have verified that the fresh fruit pulp and peel (both edible) have a strong weight loss effect and prevent the formation of new adipose cells. Ripe fruit also shown a 100% Lipase inhibitory effect (prevents the enzyme from breaking down fat in the digestive tract) which is quite impressive. Store bought fruits are too green and can be toxic. Try to find tree ripened fruit; it tastes better and has lost its toxicity.[136]

38. STEVIA (Stevia rebaudiana) – I have tried the packets and they taste terrible. But Stevioside is 100 times sweeter than sugar, so what's wrong? The packets are a standardized amount that is so small that it is worthless. I guess the billionaires want to protect their interests in all of those other CANCER-CAUSING artificial sweeteners that they also sell. The only alternative is to grow your own. You can use fresh or dried leaf and it doesn't take much to sweeten your coffee or anything else that needs a sweetener.[137]

39. SUGAR CANE (Saccharum spp.) – As bizarre as it sounds, juice of the stems (popular in Miami where it is called "Guarapo") has been shown in studies to reduce fat as well as cholesterol, despite its high sugar content, due to the many phytonutrients present in the raw juice.[138]

40. TAMARIND (Tamarindus indica) – Tamarind fruit pulp has been shown in at least one study to reduce body fat and lower LDL (the "bad") cholesterol and to elevate HDL (the "good") cholesterol. It can be found on rare occasions in the "Ethnic Foods" section of some major stores and it is highly recommended.[139]

41. TURMERIC (Curcuma longa) – This relative to Ginger has a long list of scientifically proven health benefits as well. While it has garnered a lot of attention in recent years for its potent anticancer properties, it is also a very strong anti-inflammatory that has been shown to be effective in ameliorating arthritis and it has also been shown to limit weight gain from a high fat diet. Add this strong antioxidant and Top Recommended Spice to your cooking as much as you can. It turns everything bright yellow and you can make your own yellow rice with it (turning a bad food into a good one) and add it to your own chicken soup, etc.[217]

42. WILD ALMOND (Sterculia foetida) – This rare nut has been shown to possess the ability to reduce body fat. Although the mechanism is still unknown, its effect is attributed to a unique phytochemical found in the seed called Sterculic Acid, but it also contains Malvalic Acid, Palmitic Acid, Oleic Acid and Linoleic Acid all of which have other proven health benefits as well.[218]

43. WINGED TREEBINE (Cissus quadrangularis) – A relative of the cacti, this succulent has various studies and trials showing that it can reduce fat and increase lean body mass. Products are available and do NOT overindulge and use only as directed.[140]

TOP RECOMMENDED WINGED TREEBINE SUPPLEMENT
==

MANUFACTURER: NUTRAKEY
PRODUCT NAME: Cissus Quadrangularis 120mg capsules
VENDOR WEBSITE: www.vitacost.com
VENDOR WEBPAGE: https://www.vitacost.com/nutrakey-cissus-quadrangularis-120-capsules

Vitacost appears to be planning to manufacture their own brand name products of this herb.

44. YERBA MATE (Ilex paraguariensis) – Yerba Mate is a tea made from the leaves of a South American species of Holly and is loaded with health benefits (unlike most other species of Holly that are poisonous.) Yerba Mate herbal teas are available and help curb the appetite and increase satiety (make you feel full.)[141]

RECOMMENDED YERBA MATE PRODUCT
==

MANUFACTURER: GUAYAKI
PRODUCT NAME: TRADITIONAL YERBA MATE TEA
VENDOR WEBSITE: www.vitacost.com
PRODUCT PAGE: https://www.vitacost.com/guayaki-traditional-organic-yerba-mate-tea

SATIETY

On the subject of "satiety" there are many different foods that can make you feel full (more so than others) and they have many different pathways to doing this. Those high in Dietary Fiber like Chickpeas, Lentils, Dried Plums, Oatmeal, etc and Calcium like dairy products are particularly good at making a person feel full on lower amounts of the food than other foods low in Dietary Fiber or Calcium. Non-fat Yogurt is an excellent low calorie food high in Calcium that has this effect.

CONCLUSION

The best plan is to try combinations of the above because most have unique phytonutrients and different pathways of helping to control and lose weight. The edible foods and spices should definitely all be added to your regular eating regimen because they can't hurt and they will all contribute toward the ultimate goal of making your Natural Whole Foods (Net Negative Calorie) and Holistic Herbs Diet work.

Thus far you have been armed with: the best sources of the Big 43 Essential Nutrients, 180 Net Negative Calorie Foods, and 100 plants that have specific phytonutrients that can actively promote weight loss in some way. That's a lot of information and now it is time to develop a diet constructed from all of these resources that will be highly effective at promoting weight loss.

But before you begin any diet, it is necessary to make one determination and one realization: 1) The Realization: ALL diets fail (for one reason or another) and 2) The Determination: What is the cause of your current weight? You cannot fix a problem if you cannot determine its cause. And once you realize that all diets fail and the reasons why they fail, you can then move forward with a plan that works.

THE ROOT CAUSES OF BEING OVERWEIGHT

I never liked the term "Obesity." It has a terrible sound to it in the first place and it also makes it sound like a disease. It is not a disease any more than being tall or having blond hair is a disease. It is an attribute. People who are thin are not treated like they are diseased (unless they are anorexic, of course) and no one sets out on a crusade to save the skinny people from their plight.

And this is a cultural thing. Modern society associates being skinny with being both healthy and attractive, but other cultures have not always done this. Just take a look at all of the naked women in the paintings from the Renaissance era, they are always rather "robust" because that was a sign of being able to afford to eat so it was also associated with wealth and prosperity and was therefore attractive.

The real point here is that the exact shape of a person has little to do with their health. Being far too overweight can bring poor health and being far too thin can also have serious repercussions. And both of these situations are often the result of psychological issues; what the psychologists call "Eating disorders."

And as this problem persists for years, then decades and is also repressed for years and then decades, it gets forgotten. But in the meantime the person has latched on to a lifestyle of satisfying and indeed burying the problem with "comfort food and comfort eating." I am not at all implying that this is YOUR situation but I am saying that this is prevalent in our society which is fast paced and definitely involves HIGH STRESS. And everyone has to deal with this stress and everyone deals with it in their own way. And some folks are rather adept at dealing with it and many folks are not so well equipped to deal with it.

Either way, eating a poor diet for decades can become a bad habit, as bad as any other like smoking or drinking alcohol, all of which fall under the purview of psychological symptoms of "oral fixation." And these habits are incredibly difficult to overcome because they have manifested themselves in the form of taking into the body physical substances that have definite physiological effects and the person becomes addicted to those physiological effects and when the substance is suddenly removed, the body will suffer from the physiological response known as "Withdrawal."

These symptoms are very real and can be very brutal for those trying to quit illegal drugs, but they can be just as nasty for those trying to quit drinking alcohol or cigarettes. And the body will suffer very real and brutal symptoms of withdrawal from decades of overeating as well. I know; I have been there. I quit drinking alcohol several years before I took up the challenge of quitting a poor diet and the two were comparable in their severity and difficulty, not just mentally, but physically as well.

Beating these kinds of habits involves a very real mental aspect. To quit drinking I began by replacing those deadly drinks with healthy ones. Rather than poison my fruit juices with Vodka, I just drank them without it and I stayed away from social gatherings where drinking was expected. It certainly wrecked my social life and cost me practically all of my friends at the time, but it was worth it. I cannot call anyone a friend who expects me to continue to poison myself to death.

But dealing with severe calorie restrictions is very different. I didn't overeat socially. I overindulged in food in the privacy of my own home. And unfortunately we all spend quite a lot of time in this setting – at home just a few dozen feet from the kitchen. And it was not just the amounts of the foods; it was also the food choices themselves.

How was I supposed to give up my chocolate candy bars? And my éclairs? And my "Party-sized" bags of potato chips and their requisite French onion dip? And so on. I used to joke that I was going to eat my bacon and eggs breakfast rather than a cubic inch of lettuce "until the day I die" until I realized that "the day I die" was going to be next Tuesday if I didn't do something.

At the time I had no idea that I was not just fighting a habit, and I was not just fighting the physiological response to a sudden dramatic decrease in calories, but I was also fighting millions of years of evolution. And that one is hard to beat.

You see, back in our deep dark evolutionary past we were hunter-gatherers as the anthropologists like to call them, and back then our primary objective, just like it is for animals every moment of their lives, was to fulfill the needs of the body and in order they are: Oxygen, Water, then Calories and Protein. Since breathing is not something we have to search out, then finding water would have been #1 on our ancestors' agenda. And right behind that would have been finding CALORIES. Because if you run out of fuel, then you can't find anything any more, and you starve to death; a very real concern for them, back then.

So when they did find calories, foods loaded with sugars,

starches and fats, it was mandatory to gorge on them because there were no guarantees of what they would find tomorrow. And one way to make sure that they did gorge on those high calorie foods was to find them DELICIOUS. It is no mystery why all of the modern high calorie foods are so scrumptious: evolution made sure that those who found them delicious ate the most and they were the ones who survived and we are their descendents. And that's why dough fried in pig lard and dipped in processed cane sugar is so irresistible to us today. And that is also why no one's mouth waters at the mention of Brussels sprouts or Asparagus, two foods that contain almost no sugars, starches or fats. And it is exactly the reason that potatoes, rice and corn have risen to their prominence in our culture: they are cheap and loaded with highly available starches that are quickly and easily converted to sugars in our digestive tracts.

Its already bad enough that one must fight the behavioral habit of wanting to eat while watching TV, and its that much worse having to suffer from the real withdrawal symptoms of a sudden calorie restricted diet, but to battle a million years of evolution that makes me crave every evil food and despise every good one, on top of that too? And you can bet that the food manufacturers are well aware of this. That's why they make those foods and sell them and get very rich in the process.

I can't help you with the psychological root causes behind the addiction other than to say that if you can't overcome them on your own, then seek professional help. Ignore your cultural based bias and visit a therapist. Often one session with a specialist is all a person needs to get on track.

Dealing with the physiological causes of being overweight is what this book is all about; I can definitely help you with that part of the equation. The root physiological causes are:

1) EATING THE WRONG FOODS – And by now you know what these are: "Nonfunctional Foods" that are high in calories and low in nutritional value like potatoes, rice and corn.

2) EATING TOO MUCH FOOD – This is not actually as bad as it might seem, but it is bad when all of that food is also the wrong kinds of foods. So the real problem is not "too much food" but it is actually a problem of consuming TOO MANY CALORIES. Then it is extremely bad and the two almost always go hand in hand.

3) INACTIVITY – Lack of exercise is a serious contributor to poor overall health, even for skinny folks. And it is dreadful for those who have been engaged in poor food choices in excess for far too long.

If these are the root physiological causes then the way to fix the problem is obvious: 1) Eat better foods, 2) Eat less (actually all you have to do is keep the total calories down) and 3) Exercise: to burn up the calories that you consume during the day and improve you cardiovascular system and metabolism while you are at it.

An important thing to remember is that it took many years to gain the extra weight, so losing it will also take time. I am a very impatient person, and I didn't want to spend years losing it all – I wanted it gone immediately and I did design a very effective diet for myself that worked very fast: I lost almost 60 pounds in 30 days: a feat that is generally considered IMPOSSIBLE.

One pound of human fat tissue contains 3,500 calories. If all I did was drink water and take vitamin and mineral pills, it would still take about two days to burn off one pound of fat. Eating NOTHING a person would only lose about 15 pounds per month. The person would also be starving and headed for serious health issues due to the lack of protein in particular. After one month, I had to give in to the fact that I was not getting enough of the Big 43, especially the Nine Essential Amino Acids and I had to "back down" from my extreme Net Negative Calorie Food diet and start making sure I was getting proper and complete nutrition. It took another four months to finish the task of losing a total of 120 pounds.

It is reasonable to expect to be able to lose 15 pounds per month on a diet that does not restrict your portion sizes although it will restrict your caloric intake, and you must also get all of the Big 43 essential nutrients in their proper amounts on a daily basis; this is critical to your success. It makes no sense to lose a significant amount of weight, but in doing so to also jeopardize your health.

There were a number of factors that contributed to the success of my own diet three decades ago: 1) I was young and there is a definite advantage to being young versus being a senior citizen: if I tried that diet now, I am sure it would land me in the hospital, 2) I exercised heavily every day forcing my body to dip into the fat reserves and burn them away, 3) I used the limited information science had discovered back then about the holistic powers of foods: I chose foods that were not only low in calories but that also stimulated fat burning metabolism. Without those specific phytonutrients featured prominently in my daily intake, I would not have exceeded losing half a pound per day.

I have learned a lot in the last 30 years since then. And if I were to attempt to lose that much weight now, I would do things a lot differently. For starters, I would never depend on a store-bought multivitamin: they are physically incapable of holding all of the nutrients the body needs each day. Excluding: Sulfur, Fiber, the Antioxidants and the Nine Essential Amino Acids, all of which should come from natural foods anyway, that still leaves roughly 12,125 milligrams worth of vitamins, minerals, and a few others. A multivitamin would therefore have to weigh that much to hold them all. Think about the physical size of a 500mg Vitamin C pill. A REAL multivitamin, one that would include EVERYTHING from "A to Zinc" in 100% RDA PROPER amounts would have to be the size of TWENTY-FOUR of those pills. I wouldn't want to have to swallow that thing.

Since no multivitamin CAN provide ALL of the essential nutrients in 100% RDA PROPER amounts, then none of them DO and those products are a WASTE of money and a WASTE of time. Almost all of them are loaded with synthetic forms, many of which have questionable bioavailability and safety anyway. Therefore, getting the Big 43 is not just a concern; it is a MAJOR PROBLEM for everyone, not just folks who want to lose weight, since there is no simple "One Pill Fix" for the problem.

Losing weight as rapidly as I did can put a terrible strain on the kidneys. I am sure it would cause catastrophic kidney failure if I tried to do that now. The kidneys are delicate organs and while I have found literally hundreds of holistic foods and herbs that provide protection for the liver, skin, eyes, bones, even the brain, holistic foods and herbs that provide kidney support are very RARE because the kidneys are literally very far away from the food we eat. Any nutrient that could help the kidneys must not only pass through the entire digestive tract, the phytonutrients must be absorbed and move to the liver. The liver filters these nutrients, regulates their release and modifies many of them before sending them on into the blood stream. From there the kidneys can filter them out, but they are looking for waste products. Nevertheless, they need nutrients and take their share out of the blood stream as well. But kidney supportive plants are rare and it makes no sense to jeopardize these organs and rapid weight loss definitely puts them in great danger and is simply not worth the risk.

I despise exercise. I definitely subscribe to the sedentary lifestyle. However, losing weight is a simple matter of physics. You must think of the extra pounds as what they really are: stored energy. The body has some amazing evolutionary features. One of them is that it will never throw away a single calorie. All extra calories floating around will get snatched out of the blood stream and stored by the adipose cells. Our bodies are far too efficient to let that valuable energy go to waste. So if one pound of fat tissue holds 3,500 calories, and the average person burns about 2,000 calories per day, then FASTING will take two days to burn off a single pound of fat, but ONLY if you don't exercise. Since exercise BURNS ENERGY, and fat is STORED ENERGY, then it makes sense that exercising will FORCE your body to dip into the fat reserves and burn them away.

Personally, I can't fast for thirty days, it is really hard to go just three days without eating; the body will quickly go into "Famine Shock" mode anyway. It produces chemical changes that literally lower the metabolism to conserve energy and the body also makes every effort to put the fat reserves under lock and key: to protect the adipose tissue from being used. This was all very useful a million years ago when we wandered around not knowing when we would find the next fruit tree, but it is a nuisance now when we have a reliable supply of food (the local grocery store) and NEED to actually break into the fat reserves and burn them up in order to get rid of them. Still you do have a choice. You could sit around fasting; I call this method: STARVE IN BED. It works, but for me it is far too MISERABLE. Or you could eat plenty of well chosen foods and also exercise; I call this method: MUNCH AND MARCH. They both work based on the difference between how many calories you consume each day and how many you burn. I prefer to eat every day rather than starve so exercise is the better way to go.

And I am not talking about grunting and clanging massive bar bells: that's weight training and body building. You can do that if you like, but what works even better for weight loss is aerobics. And this does not mean just walking. For aerobics to actually do something for you, the session has to reach the point in which you are breathing hard and sweating. That's when the muscles have depleted their short term anaerobic fuel supply and have to start burning sugars in the blood for fuel: the aerobic fuel supply. As the blood sugars get burned, the liver has to put more sugars back into the blood to keep the concentration at the proper level. Once the liver runs out of "sugar on hand" from your last few meals, then what? The only recourse left is to signal the adipose cells to start breaking up the fat and release it into the blood to be burned.

When the muscle cells switch to burning sugars rather than their internal anaerobic fuel supplies, the sugar has to be burned with oxygen from the air and it generates a lot more heat. This is exactly why you begin to breathe heavily, to take in the oxygen needed to burn the sugars and why you heat up and begin to sweat. Until that occurs, you are not even close to burning away your fat reserves. But once you do enter into the aerobic phase, the liver still has plenty of sugar on hand, so that must be depleted as well. Then finally, the exercise will force the body to dip into the fat reserves.

Stopping too soon is therefore useless. When you stop your exercise, the muscles immediately begin rebuilding the short-term anaerobic fuel supplies. These are what allow us to move all of the time and not have to breathe heavily and sweat while walking out to check the mail box. And once those anaerobic fuel supplies are rebuilt, then when you start to workout again, you are back to square one: forcing the muscles to exhaust this anaerobic fuel supply, then forcing the liver to give up its sugar-on-hand reserves and then finally reaching the point where the adipose cells are forced to break into their fat reserves; so one long aerobic exercise session is FAR MORE effective than many short ones. In fact, during my diet I took a long vigorous jog in the evening, lasting at about 90 minutes and sometimes ran the circuit twice.

There is no way to know how deep the liver's sugar reserves are, but the more starches and sugars you eat, the deeper those reserves will be. These are foods with high "Carb Loads" or large percentages of starches and sugars that can be used as fuel. These foods all have notoriously high Glycemic index values, foods that are bad for diabetics, and they start with the THREE MAIN FOOD CAUSES OF TYPE II DIABETES: Potatoes, Rice and Corn. Other high GI value foods are most fruits and starchy roots. By eliminating these high Carb Load foods, the liver will not have deep sugar reserves to replenish the blood sugar levels and the body will have no choice but to break into the fat reserves and that is the goal: to force the body to burn up those fat reserves. Enough with the theory, lets get to the details.

THE EFFECTIVE DIET PLAN – PRE-DIET PREP

1. ADAPTOGENS – No matter what you do, the body will notice the sudden drop in caloric intake and it will respond with "Famine Shock" mode, severely lowering the metabolism and protecting the fat reserves. That has to be thwarted before it even begins. One of the most effective adaptogens for stabilizing hormone levels that accompany Famine Shock is ELEUTHERO ROOT. It is available from many different vendors; get at least a thirty day supply and begin taking it at least a few days before the actual diet – calorie restrictions – begin. If you want to include other adaptogens from the list, add them one at a time after at least a two day start on the first one to make sure that you do not have an adverse reaction to any of them. So you would start your daily dose of Eleuthero root on Sunday, followed by starting a daily dose of Jiaogulan on Tuesday, Dong Quai on Thursday, etc. Eleuthero alone should be sufficient but since every person is different, it might not be as effective for you, so using two or three might be the way to go. I really wish I had known about Eleuthero back when I tried several times to diet; it would have prevented my body from entering Famine Shock mode causing me to gain weight while suffering through one commercial diet after another.

2. GET THE BIG 43 – You must get these squared away before you really start the caloric restrictions. Failing to get the essential nutrients will put your body on high alert and it will resist the diet primarily with cravings for your favorite foods. This is largely due to the sudden reduction in calories, but also the body is calling for essential nutrients that have suddenly disappeared from your diet as well. By providing everything the body needs, then it won't need to raise the alarm: so it won't hit you with cravings as much. Since multivitamins, especially store-bought brands, are USELESS, INSUFFICIENT, and made with INFERIOR QUALITY SYNTHETIC ingredients, here is everything you need.

A. COD LIVER OIL (1teaspoon/day, **41 cal**) – Vitamin A, Vitamin D3, 888mg Omega-3 DHA and EPA.

B. YEAST EXTRACT SPREAD ("Vegemite" 1oz/day, **44 cal**) – Vitamins B1, B2, and B3, plus 71% B9.

C. B VITAMIN SUPPLEMENTS: You could take an individual supplement for VITAMIN B5 – PANTOTHENIC ACID,

VITAMIN B6 - PYRIDOXINE, and VITAMIN B7 – BIOTIN, all of which force you to assemble lists of foods to eat throughout the day to make sure you get them in proper amounts and those foods are loaded with fat, cholesterol and calories, or you could take a single high quality Vitamin B Complex made from natural extract sources of all eight of the B Vitamins and that provides them all in at least 100% RDA amounts.

D. CABBAGE (1 cup/day, **35 cal**) – This Net Negative Calorie food is a superior side dish for dinner, it brings more VITAMIN C than any Citrus fruit and is loaded with Glucosinolates – SULFUR-containing compounds – that bring a wide range of health benefits.

E. GRAPEFRUIT (3 per day, **300cal**) – This Net Negative Calorie fruit will provide you with plenty of VITAMIN C and the Grapefruit brings Synephrine which stimulates fat burning metabolism (it was a significant reason why my diet worked.)

F. VITAMIN E SUPPLEMENT – The only natural sources are seeds and nuts which bring a ton of calories.

TOP RECOMMENDED VITAMIN E SUPPLEMENTS
==

MANUFACTURER: JARROW FORMULAS
PRODUCT NAME: FAMIL-E
WEBSITE: www.jarrow.com
PRODUCT PAGE: www.jarrow.com/product/292/Famil-E
==

MANUFACTURER: NOW FOODS
PRODUCT NAME: VITAMIN E 200 IU MIXED
  TOCOPHEROLS SOFTGELS
WEBSITE: www.nowfoods.com
PRODUCT PAGE: www.nowfoods.com/supplements/vitamin-
  e-200-iu-mixed-tocopherols-softgels
==

MANUFACTURER: Dr. MERCOLA
PRODUCT NAME: MERCOLA VITAMIN E
WEBSITE: www.mercola.com
PRODUCT PAGE: https://products.mercola.com/vitamine/

You do not have to follow my recommendation but, all three of these include many different forms of Vitamin E and from natural sources.

G. KALE (1oz/day, **14 cal**) – Tossed into the lunch salad this will bring plenty of VITAMIN K as well as Lutein and Zeaxanthin; powerful antioxidants that promote liver, skin and eye health.

H. YOGURT (2cups/day, **300 cal**) – Yogurt is relatively low calorie and provides Calcium in a natural form which is far superior to any pill. If you are lactose intolerant and cannot eat diary products, you will have to find a high quality calcium supplement like Calcium Citrate. It should be 500mg twice a day.

I. CHOLINE SUPPLEMENT – This nutrient is only found in significant quantities in foods very high in saturated fat and cholesterol. While on your diet you will definitely need to take a Choline supplement; it is critical for proper liver and BRAIN function.

TOP RECOMMENDED CHOLINE SUPPLEMENTS
==

MANUFACTURER: NOW FOODS
PRODUCT NAME: CHOLINE & INOSITOL, 500 MG, 100 CAPSULES
WEBSITE: www.nowfoods.com
PRODUCT PAGE: www.nowfoods.com/supplements/choline-inositol-500-mg-capsules
==

MANUFACTURER: NOW FOODS
PRODUCT NAME: ALPHA GPC, 300 MG, 60 CAPSULES
WEBSITE: www.nowfoods.com
PRODUCT PAGE: www.nowfoods.com/supplements/alpha-gpc-300-mg-veg-capsules

You could get away with alternating these two (one a day, the first on Monday, the alpha-GPC on Tuesday, etc) which can help offset the high price of the Alpha-GPC, but don't scrimp, it is expensive from any vendor and is a form already proven capable of passing across the blood-brain barrier much more readily than any other.

10) BROCCOLI (steamed 1.5 cup/day, **82 cal**) – Chromium is a real problem. If you are serious about this diet, you should actually plan on eating about 1.5 cups of steamed Broccoli every day. That will bring all of the Chromium you need along with more Vitamin C and Vitamin K.

TOP RECOMMENDED CHROMIUM SUPPLEMENT
==

MANUFACTURER: JARROW FORMULAS
PRODUCT NAME: CHROMIUM GTF, 200 MCG, 100 CAPS
WEBSITE: www.jarrow.com
PRODUCT PAGE: www.jarrow.com/product/214/Chromium_GTF

This product provides Chromium as a chelate believed to be superior to Chromium Picolinate. Many health professionals are questioning the picolinate and suspect that it might be CARCINOGENIC. It's in almost all store-bought brands and not worth the risk. This product provides about three times the Consensus Daily Value which means you could take one pill every other day to help offset the expense.

J. OYSTERS (canned, 2oz twice per week, **39 cal/serving**) – They are low calorie and will bring all the ZINC you need and plenty of COPPER as well. For those who do not want to eat oysters a dedicated high quality supplement is a must.

TOP RECOMMENDED ZINC SUPPLEMENTS

===

MANUFACTURER: NOW FOODS
PRODUCT NAME: L-OPTIZINC 30 MG
WEBSITE: www.nowfoods.com
PRODUCT PAGE: www.nowfoods.com/supplements/
l-optizinc-30-mg-veg-capsules

===

MANUFACTURER: GARDEN OF LIFE
PRODUCT NAME: VITAMIN CODE RAW ZINC
WEBSITE: www.gardenoflife.com
PRODUCT PAGE: www.gardenoflife.com/content/product/
vitamin-code-raw-zinc/

K. CLAMS (6.5oz can, twice per week, **270 cal/serving**) – They will bring you the majority of the IRON you need plus a little COPPER as well. They will also bring you a total of 6,000% VITAMIN B12 for the week. No harm in loading up on a safe water-soluble BRAIN nutrient.

L. SEA SALT (½ teaspoon/day) – This covers SODIUM, CHLORINE and IODINE.

M. MILK OF MAGNESIA (2 teaspoons/day) – Take one teaspoon at a time at the midpoint between meals. Because it neutralizes stomach acid and will interfere with digestion, do not take it prior to, during, or immediately after eating. It will provide all of your MAGNESIUM for the day.

N. OATS (old-fashioned, precooked, ½ cup/day, **150 cal**) – The Oats will bring half of your MANGANESE and MOLYBDENUM along with BETA-GLUCANS which are immunostimulants and have proven anticancer properties.

O. BANANAS (10oz, 2 large fruits per day, **250 cal**) – The Bananas will bring 30% of both DIETARY FIBER and POTASSIUM.

P. BRAZIL NUTS (2 nuts/day, **80 cal**) – These have the highest concentration of SELENIUM of any food on Earth. Think of them as tasty chewable natural Selenium supplements.

Q. ONIONS/LEEKS/SCALLIONS (1.25 cup/day, **115 cal**) – These foods are loaded with SULFUR compounds that bring a wide range of health benefits. Raw chopped onions should be left to "breathe" for a few minutes before eating them to allow a detrimental chemical to disintegrate. All three are perfectly safe after any amount of cooking.

R. LOW SODIUM ORIGINAL V-8 (16oz/day, **90 cal**) – This will bring about 56% RDA POTASSIUM and it is very low calorie.

S. OMEGA-3 DHA/EPA SUPPLEMENT – Take at least 500mg per day in addition to the O3FA's you get from the COD LIVER OIL. Any reputable brand is fine.

T. GREEN PEAS, CHICKPEAS, LENTILS, BLACK BEANS (1 cup every other day, **117 cal** for canned Green Peas) – These bring MOLYBDENUM, and a lot of DIETARY FIBER. The LENTILS (230cal/cup) and BLACK BEANS (218 cal/cup) bring about 2/3 of your daily DIETARY FIBER and are also loaded with ANTIOXIDANTS. LENTILS bring 90% VITAMIN B9 – FOLATE and CHICKPEAS (269 cal/cup) bring 71%.

U. DRIED PLUMS (1 cup every other day, **418 cal/serving**) – The cup of Prunes is for the days that you skip the above legumes. They bring 50% DIETARY FIBER and 36% POTASSIUM.

V. FISH (5oz/day, **162 cal for Tuna**) – TUNA, SALMON, COD, MACKEREL, SARDINES, etc. These five are all excellent sources of Complete Protein (they bring all Nine of the Essential Amino Acids in reasonable amounts and proportions and help you to keep your total amount of protein DOWN along with bringing very little Saturated Fat. Most seeds and Nuts actually have more Saturated Fat in them than any Fish. The fish do bring Cholesterol, but relying on plants for Complete Protein will force you to eat a lot more. It would take 40 oz of Avocado to match the amounts of all nine essential amino acids in 5 ounces of any Fish. That's about 1,800 calories. And it would take at least 1,000 calories worth of nuts to accomplish that as well so for now, stick to the fish. They also bring more of the almighty Omega-3 Fatty Acids DHA and EPA anyway.

This is an excellent head start on not only getting all of the Big 43 but also in getting a whole host of benefits from the various natural constituents in these foods. The total calories for those items to be consumed daily is about 1,580 calories, so you will still have to make some choices about which ones to replace with high quality supplements.

3. EXERCISE – Get this rolling before you start reducing your daily caloric intake. You must ease into exercise if you are not used to it. It makes no sense to jump onto an exercise bicycle for several hours and end up in the Emergency Room. Gradually increase your aerobic workout each day until you can reach a point where you are breathing heavily and sweating and can maintain that for at least one hour per day. This should take you a few weeks. Once you are at this level, then the real diet can begin.

THE EFFECTIVE NATURAL WHOLE FOOD DIET
FOR LOSING WEIGHT BEGINS NOW

1. SUBSTITUTE THE SNACKS – The only items allowed for snacks are Net Negative Calorie foods. Within them there are two extremely effective foods: Celery, which is a triple play for the diet:

it is an Adaptogen, a Diuretic, and a Net Negative Calorie food. Do not underestimate its power to help you lose weight; it was a key component of my diet. It works. You can literally eat as much of it as you want throughout the day. I know it is not tasty and do NOT be tempted to sprinkle it with salt or use any dip or salad dressing. Think of it as a power tool that will actively participate in helping you to shed weight fast. Other great low calorie snacks include Cucumbers, Pickles, Carrots, etc. Be wary of store-bought pickles, they add sugars that make their caloric value and Glycemic Index values soar through the roof. If you cannot find pickles below 4 cal/oz then make your own. Slice your cucumbers (they pickle faster when sliced) and place them in a clean jar. 2) Fill half way with White vinegar, 3) Add about ½ teaspoon of Turmeric powder (this is the original healthy formula for making them yellow) 1 Tbsp of dill weed, and any other spices you might like (I add 1 Tbsp each of minced garlic, oregano and black peppercorns) 4) Seal the jar and shake it up, 5) Finish filling the jar with Red Wine Vinegar to get in on the powerful phytonutrients of grapes and the sweeter taste, 6) Throw the jar into the back of the refrigerator for a few months, 7) Serve your own healthy delicious pickles.

2. TRANSFORM BREAKFAST – It should be nothing but ½ cup (precooked) Old-Fashioned Oatmeal for the duration of the diet and beyond. Sweeten it with a little Raw Bee Honey or even better use fresh STEVIA LEAVES. The packets have too little Stevia in them and are very expensive and do not sweeten anything to my liking, but fresh Stevia leaves are very sweet and it won't take much to do the trick. You can also add Raisins, "Craisins" (dried Cranberries) sliced Bananas, Apples, etc. In addition, have one whole Grapefruit; peel and eat like an Orange and do NOT garnish it with sugar. Accompany breakfast with an 8 ounce cup of Campbell Soup Company Brand LOW SODIUM ORIGINAL V-8 (Yes, I wish I owned some stock!)

3. TRANSFORM LUNCH – This should be a tossed salad for the rest of the diet and beyond. A bowl of chopped lettuce with a pinch of fresh Kale, chopped Onion (let it sit for 5 minutes to dissipate a detrimental chemical that forms when they are chopped) sliced Cucumbers, etc is very nutritious and very low calorie. Oil and Vinegar dressing should be the only one you use for the rest of your life. The creamy dressings are made from raw eggs that block the absorption of Vitamin B7 – Biotin which is extremely difficult to get from natural whole foods and you will likely be paying for supplements to get it, so you can't AFFORD to eat Mayonnaise or its kin. You can certainly make your own Oil and Vinegar dressing. It's easy: Pour one pint of Extra Virgin Olive Oil into a large clean jar then add two tablespoons of Red Wine Vinegar, then you can add Spices to your heart's content. I add a tablespoon each of Oregano, Parsley, Cilantro, Black Peppercorns, Minced Onions and Minced Garlic. You also do not have to stick strictly to Extra

Virgin Olive Oil either. You could start with Safflower Oil (#1 all-purpose oil) or Canola. You could then add a few tablespoons of the Olive Oil, and/or Sesame Seed Oil, Extra Virgin Coconut Oil, or even Borage Oil (very high in Conjugated Linoleic Acid (a very effective anti-inflammatory that promotes weight-loss too) or even Peanut Oil for the remarkable taste, or Avocado Oil for those unusual monounsaturated fats and Medium Chain Triglycerides. Accompany your salad with an 8 ounce cup of Yogurt and an 8 ounce cup of Campbell Soup Company Brand LOW SODIUM ORIGINAL V-8. You can try another brand, but read the Nutrition Label and make sure it brings at least 20% of the RDA amount of POTASSIUM.

4. TRANSFORM DINNER – Dinner is wide open, but at least two nights a week it should be New England Clam Chowder. If you don't know how to make it, do this: 1) Pour 1 can of Ready-to-Eat New England Clam Chowder into a pot, 2) Add 1 can Condensed New England Clam Chowder, 3) Add one 6.5oz can of Chopped Clams liquid and all, 4) Add 2oz of canned Boiled Oysters. Stir while heating and serve. I also throw in a can of boiled Spinach and a heaping teaspoon each of Black Pepper, Minced Garlic, Cilantro, Parsley and Oregano. It turns green, but it's delicious and packed with antioxidants and many powerful phytonutrients. The other nights, 5 ounces of any Fish should be the entrée and only baked. Sides should come from the Net Negative Calorie foods list and there are literally over a hundred to choose from, so you shouldn't get bored! If you don't know how to cook, then "No Salt Added" canned goods are fine. But they are overcooked and have lost a lot of their nutritional value especially the antioxidants.

5) CONCENTRATE ON THE NET NEGATIVE CALORIE FOODS – Always look to substitute foods that are high in calories with foods that are much lower in calories and that also bring with them useful nutrition. Even though the serving size might not fulfill your daily requirement of Vitamin K, Watercress is still an outstanding vegetable that can be added to soups, stews, salads, etc that adds to the portion size or VOLUME of the meal while only adding 3.7 calories per cup. The major purpose of these foods is not simply their nutritional value even though some are true superfoods like raw Kale, Swiss Chard and steamed or boiled Collard Greens, but because they allow you to consume much larger portion sizes in your meals which helps alleviate the anxiety caused by a calorie restricted diet. While I was very willing to "tough it out" it is still MISERABLE and by being able to eat unlimited amounts of the Net Negative Calorie foods this helped to alleviate the constant feeling of hunger and cravings for those old terrible high calorie foods that I had become accustomed to eating for years.

6) DON'T FORGET THE DIETARY FIBER-RICH FOODS – These foods definitely help with Satiety. They are very filling and make you feel full for a much longer period of time afterwards which is a great help in curbing the urge to snack. Dietary Fiber promotes intestinal health and sticks to cholesterol preventing its absorption in the digestive tract; all three of these benefits are EXCELLENT for your health and can go a long way toward helping you with the diet plan.

7) SEEK OUT ANTIOXIDANTS – Many of these natural whole foods have also shown significant anti-inflammatory properties as well as relieving "oxidative stress." This not only improves your health, it actually makes you FEEL much better and that can go a long way toward encouraging anyone to stick to a diet.

8) EMPTY THE SPICE RACK – On the subject of Antioxidants and Anti-inflammatory properties, the Spices are definitely loaded with both. If you want to put down the BB gun and pick up a HOWITZER of health promoting benefits, then the Spices are the Big Guns you want. Even with canned goods you can add a teaspoon of Oregano, or Marjoram (a close relative that has a much more delicate aroma and flavor) or fresh Basil. I add a teaspoon of Clove powder to my weekly Chili (made with lean Ground Turkey.) You can still taste it but the fresh Jalapeños and Cayenne pepper help to hide it and Clove powder does have one of the highest ORAC Scores of anything you will find at your local grocery store; a whopping 290,283.

9) ADD THE HOLISTIC FOODS AND SPICES – Add as many edible plant foods that bring helpful properties for your effort – I have listed as many as I could find and I am sure that there are many more. Since many of these foods are also Net Negative Calorie foods as well then they should be the top priority foods to substitute into your regular dietary regimen. Like all STRONG MEDICINE; MORE IS NEVER BETTER. So use the "Shotgun" approach and add as many DIFFERENT holistic foods as you can in reasonable portion sizes rather than overdoing it on just one or a few. This will prevent you from overdosing on the phytonutrients they contain and at the same time add to the array of tools that are working to help you achieve your goal. The more weapons you bring to the fight, the greater your chances of winning the fight.

10) ADD THE HOLISTIC HERBS – You can try Diuretics if you need them, but remember that Black Pepper and Celery have this effect and are much safer than any supplement so see if they work before adding stronger diuretics. You can add more metabolism boosters, but dessert for each meal should be a whole grapefruit – they are very low calorie and the Synephrine is very effective. You can add herbs with appetite suppression properties, but Yogurt (high in Calcium) and all of the high Dietary Fiber foods increase Satiety – they make you feel fuller faster and make that feeling last longer and are a top priority. After Eleuthero root, you can add a few more of the Adaptogens too. Just remember that you must not overindulge in any single holistic herb, especially in supplement form; the goal is to get BETTER, NOT WORSE.

The Natural Whole Foods Diet has to be modified for those who wish to lose weight basically by removing the seeds and nuts which are too high in calories to be practical.

But before you do anything else, you must make sure that you are getting the Big 43 Essential Nutrients in at least the 100% RDA amounts daily. The two notable exceptions to this rule are Vitamin C which should be taken in larger amounts than the paltry 60mg that the FDA recommends and Sulfur which has no established RDA, but the simple sulfur compounds present in garlic, onions, leeks, etc. are of enormous health value and must be included in your regular eating regimen.

While regularly checking your car's fluids and tire pressure won't make it fly, it will improve gas mileage and help make trips to the mechanic's shop less frequent. The exact same thing is true of the human body. By providing it with everything it needs in the proper amounts, it will function better and result in fewer trips to the doctor's office too.

We only need 6 mcg (micrograms) of Vitamin B12 daily which is literally a microscopic amount. But that still contains trillions of molecules, enough for each brain cell to get some and that's the organ that depends on it. Without it, the brain – YOU-the-person – begins to malfunction and that can have terrible consequences for YOU-the-person including anxiety, depression, short-term memory loss, etc. Modern life is already filled with enough events and situations that can cause all of these terrible psychological effects without fanning the flames by missing out not only on those simple 6mcg of Vitamin B12, but ALL of the rest of the B Vitamins and indeed all of the rest of the Big 43.

Knowing what the body needs and how to fulfill those needs is imperative and it certainly doesn't stop at the Big 43, rather it starts there. But if the Big 43 have not been taken care of, then nothing else you try to do will work.

In the long term, popping pills to get at least 34 of those essential nutrients (excluding the 9 essential amino acids which can be taken care of with about 5 ounces of any Complete protein animal meat) will not work either. We spent millions of years evolving and consuming mostly (about 90% daily average) edible raw plants and each one of them provides not only calories (fuel) and proteins (construction material for new cells in all organs) but also some of the recognized Big 43 essential nutrients as well as HUNDREDS of other phytonutrients and trace minerals that the body also needs.

If the FDA takes decades to evaluate the results of numerous scientific research studies to determine a useful Recommended Daily Allowance for even the most critical essential nutrients, it would take them several thousand years to establish the RDA's of all of those other phytonutrients in just ONE plant that most health professionals are certain that we also need. Granted, we might not need all of them from a single plant, but most plants bring a few and even dozens that already have the studies backing up the fact that they do have measurable health benefits and the established RDA's for the few substances that we do know to be essential are often conservative, especially the water soluble vitamins, with Vitamin C being the noteworthy example.

As for the minerals, you should try not to exceed the RDA amounts because in excess most can become TOXIC. Even Iron, as critical as it is to human life, can become TOXIC in excess and cause serious trouble for the liver.

Others like Choline in particular are very difficult to establish a "one size fits all" amount because different people have different requirements of this critical nutrient involved in brain function as well as a host of other functions throughout the body.

To make matters even more confusing, many members of the "Big 43" come in different forms. Vitamin A is Retinol, a diterpenoid (20 carbon atoms in its molecular skeleton,) while beta-Carotene is a tetraterpenoid (40 carbon atoms in its molecular skeleton.) The body can easily convert beta-Carotene into Vitamin A as needed by literally snapping it in half like a wishbone yielding a Retinol molecule, but we do not know if the body can keep up with the demand for Vitamin A with this process leading many health professionals to the conclusion that we still need to get some "true" Vitamin A as Retinol on a daily basis. Vitamin E from natural sources, mostly seeds and nuts, comes in at least eight different compounds collectively called Tocopherols and Tocotrienols. We still do not know the specific amounts of each one that we need and we can be certain that they all have slightly different functions that could end up being very significant in the long run if any one of them is missing from a person's intake for years at a time.

There is sufficient evidence that we also need Inositol, a molecular relative of Choline and the rest of the B Vitamins. And it may turn out that certain Omega-6 Fatty Acids are as essential to human health as the Omega-3's for which the FDA is planning to set an RDA (the first RDA to be established in years, by the way.) And despite the hype about them, every health professional on the planet strongly advocates including as many antioxidant-rich foods as you can into your daily diet. Does this mean they are essential nutrients too? Beta-Carotene could certainly be considered an essential nutrient, especially for those who do not get any true Vitamin A as Retinol in their diet on a daily basis and it is an antioxidant of great importance for eye and skin health and is about 25 times more potent than Vitamin C.

Evidence suggests that communities and cultures with high antioxidant-rich diets have longer average life expectancies than communities and cultures with relatively poor antioxidant intake.

And those communities and cultures with the antioxidant-rich diets experience far lower rates of high blood pressure, high cholesterol, diabetes, cardiovascular disease and cancer. Those five maladies are reaching epidemic proportions in the U.S. and heart failure (almost always the result of chronic cardiovascular disease) and cancer together are now responsible for 1.24 MILLION deaths each year and that number is rising every year. It would seem that the statistics support the conclusion that antioxidants are as essential to human health as any of the other essential nutrients like the Omega-3 Fatty Acids.

And we are always discovering new phytonutrients and just as importantly, the specific health benefits of countless known ones every year. Some blow up and turn into fad plants or supplements and quite often they are very well deserving of the notice, but too often such crazes pass and the population jumps onto the next one that comes along. Obviously, the plant didn't suddenly lose its beneficial properties, just the attention it was getting.

To that end, the most important thing to remember is to ignore the hype and forget about the modern fixation on "one quick pill cures" because for the most part those are pipe dreams anyway. Reaching OPTIMUM THRIVE-LEVEL health and MAINTAINING it is work, plain and simple. But it is not as bad as stacking 80lb bags of concrete for 16 hours every day. Aside from a very beneficial hour of aerobics daily, the work is very simple: know what your body needs for optimum health and then give it what it needs.

As for losing weight, the formula is also simple: eliminate fast food and junk food, eliminate high calorie, high cholesterol foods, eliminate "nonfunctional foods" (those that have low nutritional or medicinal value) and replace them all with the Net Negative Calorie foods and Functional Foods; those that are high in nutritional and/or medicinal value, and add herbal teas and/or supplements that will actively support your effort and don't forget that aerobic exercise; it is vital to achieving and maintaining OPTIMUM THRIVE-LEVEL health and well-being.

The preceding chapters have lined up 58 Superfoods that can bring the Big 43 essential nutrients in reasonable serving sizes, but not necessarily convenient caloric content. Also included in that list are the best supplements for getting those essential nutrients when the foods are either unavailable or too high in calories.

The next chapter included a list of 180 Net Negative Calorie foods plus four more low calorie foods that bring Complete Protein, many of which are also Superfoods or Functional foods that bring either high nutrient content or holistic health benefits or both. There are enough foods in that list that a person could construct a sufficiently varied weekly dietary regimen out of them and only need to add oatmeal and of course the spices and be set up not only with a healthy and nutritious diet, but also one very well suited to losing weight easily.

The following chapters empowered you with over 100 holistic foods, spices and medicinal herbs (counting the many different edible mushrooms) that can and will provide the necessary added natural support for any serious weight loss effort. These are like the free agents acquired by a professional sports team that can provide enough help to win the championship. By themselves, they can't get you to optimum health or immediately to your target weight, but without them it would take a lot longer and be a lot more miserable along the way.

The Net Negative Calorie foods should be the majority of the foods you eat throughout the day, add into the mix two different stimulants (not just tons of caffeine) and add in sources of appetite suppressants, others that block the production of adipose cells, those that increase fat metabolism and most importantly add more than one adaptogen; plants that help the body deal with stress and inhibit the production of hormonal responses to a diet based on a reduction in caloric intake.

BEST PRACTICES

1. HAVE A PLAN – The plan is to transform your daily dietary regimen for the rest of your life, You do not want to "go on a diet" in order to suffer through it to finally reach your target weight, then relax and end up where you started.

2. START WITH THE HOLISTIC HERBS – At the very least you should begin by taking Eleuthero and perhaps another one of the adaptogens well-suited for weight loss. Throw in a couple effective metabolism boosters like Grapefruit and Cinnamon. Two great appetite suppressants are Fennel and Gamboge. Etc.

3. REPLACE THE BAD WITH THE GOOD – Start with snacks. I snack often and by replacing chips and dip, cookies, etc. with low calorie alternatives like celery this resulted in an immediate and drastic reduction in daily caloric intake (by THOUSANDS of calories per day) as well as a huge improvement in overall health by adding the antioxidant power of these foods and the holistic power of the celery.

4. TRANSFORM ONE MEAL AT A TIME – Breakfast is the easiest one to change. It should be oatmeal and add a tablespoon of Wheat Germ. Add sliced fresh fruits and sweeten with Raw Bee Honey or Stevia (the packets are terrible, it doesn't take much fresh leaf Stevia to make the bowl sweet.) Lunch is also easy: it should be a tossed salad adorned with Oil and Vinegar dressing. For dinner replace the rice, corn, potatoes and other nonfunctional side dishes with an assortment of the Net Negative Calorie foods, Even 8 ounces of many of the fish in the Net Negative Calorie foods list will still bring far fewer calories than most other land animal meats mainly because they are all very low in Saturated Fat (it must be from always running away from the bigger fish!)

and they are far better for you because they all have some of the
Omega-3 Fatty Acids DHA and EPA in them.

5. HUNT FOR BETTER CHOICES – It is an ongoing process.
Always be on the lookout for beneficial supplements, herbal teas
(which usually bring no few calories and loads of health boosting
phytonutrients) spices (that are powerhouses of antioxidants and
holistic phytonutrients) and fresh fruits and vegetables (also very
low calorie with high nutritional and holistic content.) Many folks
get "stuck in a flavor rut" and don't like to try new foods. I was like
that but now I am the opposite; I am eager to try new foods and
many turn out to be exquisite. I have run into my share of foods I
don't like very much as well, but that is what garlic, onions, bell
peppers and the spices were invented for: to repair a food's flavor
and if that doesn't work, then they can overwhelm it.

6. DON'T SWEAT THE DETAILS – If you stick to the plan and
replace high calorie foods with the Net Negative Calorie foods then
you will lose weight. I am not an advocate of counting calories
unless you really want to do that. But having boiled spinach and
green peas as my sides for dinner, I know they don't add up to
much, so a second helping of both will not take me way over the
top: and that is the key to sticking with the Net Negative Calorie
foods. They make staying fit easy and fun because you don't have
to always run to the nutrition label and calculate how many
calories are in the serving you want to eat. When it comes to
skinned cucumbers, you can eat them until you can't eat any
more, and still probably haven't passed a few dozen calories
worth. And when dieting in this way you don't have to jump on the
scale every five minutes either because it isn't necessary and just
adds more stress which is always a bad idea. Trust the Net
Negative Calorie foods and a nice spread of holistic herbs to do
their jobs and they will deliver the desired results.

LAST THOUGHTS

You certainly do not have to include any of the Superfoods that
bring significant amounts of some of members of the Big 43 like
Clams or Oysters. But if you do skip any of them, be sure to
include high quality supplements, preferably those that are based
on natural food source extracts rather than synthetics.

Dieting is all about PHYSICS; to lose weight you must BURN
OFF more calories than you consume each day. The wider this
margin, the faster you will lose those extra unwanted pounds. The
"Starve in Bed" method is too miserable to put up with and it is
completely unnecessary and it is far less effective than the "Munch
and March" method anyway. The more work you do throughout the
day, the more calories you burn, far more than just sitting around
starving. By losing almost TWO POUNDS each day, that means
that I must have been burning about six thousand calories during
my evening runs and I assure you I was exhausted when I got

home, but it was worth it both for losing the weight and improving my cardiovascular health.

Now that I am much older, I would definitely ease into that much exercise and probably would never reach that level of exercise, but I would still put forth the effort, as much effort as possible. So whatever you can do, it is infinitely better than doing nothing at all.

The main objections to the Natural Whole Foods Diet are: 1) It's too expensive, 2) It takes too much planning, 3) Don't know how to cook, 4) Studies are done with concentrated extracts and mostly on mice so they are not "Real World" applicable, 5) Grocery store produce is covered in pesticides which are just as toxic as the additives in packaged foods, and 6) A Natural Whole Foods diet consisting primarily of Net Negative Calorie Foods doesn't taste as good.

I have known many people who eat very well – proper Natural Whole Food diets – on Food Stamps. I am not suggesting a diet of Live Maine Lobster and Filet Mignon every night. I am suggesting simply to pay closer attention to the amounts of Nonfunctional foods loaded with trash calories and little nutritional or medicinal value in your diet and replace the bad foods with good ones. A can of No Salt added Green Peas rather than Pinto beans literally costs no extra and as you go through making such replacements in every meal, they add up to a far superior regular eating regimen that can literally save your life.

As for the planning, this book has laid out everything you need to get the Big 43 plus almost two hundred low calorie foods and 110 holistic foods, spices and herbs that act directly within the body to assist with weight loss. The idea was not to overload you with information but to provide you with plenty of alternatives to choose from that can and will help you achieve your goal.

As for cooking skill, I assure that I started out incapable of boiling water or frying an egg. Even now I would not call myself a "Chef" but it doesn't take much skill or time (about 15 minutes) to boil a pot of sliced yellow squash (a great NNC Food) either. It does take a little time to learn how to cook some foods and I wasted half a bag of dried lentils before I got the hang of cooking them, but it was well worth the effort: they have an ORAC score of over 7,000 making them TEN TIMES stronger in antioxidant power than raw carrots.

As for the studies being done with concentrated extracts and usually being done on mice and not men, the issue is complicated. I can say that mice are a lot closer to us than anyone would care to admit and usually what is good for them is good for us and what is bad for them is bad for us and vice versa. Studies on mice often use concentrated extracts, but they also subject them to highly exaggerated issues for the plant extract to counteract (such as a diet consisting of almost nothing but animal fat) and because the studies cannot take years, but usually just a few weeks or months, the studies must show a measurable result quickly. So while the positive effects of the plant extract are measurable within a month of two while subjecting mice to a very high saturated fat diet, if a person reduces this as much as possible and includes the plant regularly in their own diet, it will help, not in a few weeks perhaps, but it will have a positive effect in the long run.

As for the pesticides on produce, you can certainly spend more money on the Organic Produce and in most cases they are far superior and have no trace of pesticides or fungicides in them. But in the end, the only way to be fair is to say that both fresh produce and packaged and processed foods all contain known toxins. If that is an unavoidable evil of all foods, then the only comparison left is the actual foods themselves. Since packaged and processed foods have low nutritional or medicinal content and tons of calories, while Natural Whole Foods have much higher nutritional and medicinal content with lower calories then those are the superior choices. And many natural foods like Red Delicious Apples are so loaded with powerful antioxidants that they literally help protect your body from those poisons while the packaged and processed cookies, chips, etc have almost no antioxidants in them and expose you to the full effects of their added chemical poisons.

As for taste, that is a matter of perspective. There is no way to defend the taste of Cod Liver Oil, but it is also really just a natural supplement. And while Oatmeal is rather bland on its own, you can certainly dress it up with spices like Nutmeg or ground Cinnamon as well as fresh sliced fruit like bananas. In the end, you will have to decide for yourself which foods you prefer: high calorie and low nutritional value packaged and processed foods that are designed to be delicious so you will get addicted to them and spend your money on them, or low calorie and high nutritional and medicinal value foods that come from nature and provide far superior health. I wouldn't write home about the majority of them as far as their taste, but because they are much better for my health and reduce the risks of some if not all of the BIG SEVEN modern deadly epidemic plagues, they taste very good to me!

THANK YOU AND GOD BLESS AND GOOD LUCK AND ABOVE ALL ELSE: TAKE CARE OF YOURSELF! (BECAUSE NO ONE ELSE IS GOING TO DO IT)

SOURCES OF INFORMATION
ANNIE'S REMEDY
WEBSITE: www.anniesremedy.com

A valuable online source of information with well over 300 plants listed in their database which was instrumental in the writing of this book. They also sell high quality Essential Oils.

Dr. Godofredo Stuart, Jr. M.D.
WEBSITE: www.stuartxchange.org

This is one of the largest databases of medicinal plants (800+ plants) on the Internet and a valuable tool without which I would not have been able to write this book.

THE FDA and the NIH
U.S. Food and Drug Administration: www.fda.gov
National Institutes for Health: www.nih.gov

Both of these governmental agencies have informative websites. Like all governmental agencies, their websites can be difficult to navigate and much of the material is either too simplified or too complicated to be of much value, but I still recommend that you visit them and take a look around.

Dr. James Duke's Phytochemical & Ethnobotanical Database
WEBSITE: https://phytochem.nal.usda.gov/phytochem/search/list

Kept at the USDA's website, this has the detailed chemical analysis of over 2,000 plants. Finding some constituents of foods like Iodine can be difficult, but if the plant is in this database then the amount in the plant will be included in the analysis.

"DR. AXE"
WEBSITE: www.draxe.com

Josh Axe has an extensive website which I have used as a primary base source of most of the information on the essential nutrients, whole foods health benefits, and unbiased reports on many supplements, that includes excellent explanations of the health benefits of each one, the nasty results of chronic deficiency for each one, and a list of foods that contain them. The website covers a lot of ground too, not just the "ABC's" (the vitamins and minerals) but also many other health food items and supplements like Lycopene, Milk Thistle, and fad products like Creatine, etc.

"MY FOOD DATA"
WEBSITE: www.myfooddata.com

This is another superb website although they don't get too deep into the nature of each nutrient and it is far from complete like "Dr. Axe" but they do have excellent lists of the top foods that contain each essential nutrient that they do cover and it is a good source of that specific information and I highly recommend that you check it out too.

THE GEORGE MATELJAN FOUNDATION
WEBSITE: www.whfoods.org

This is one of the best reference websites that covers many minerals in excellent detail that most other websites do not. They include a lot of good information on the function of most of the nutrients in the body as well, some of which I could only find at this website and I could never have written this book without their vast collection of nutritional information. They include a lot of additional and useful information about the individual natural whole foods including recipes and weekly diet plans. Check it out.

WIKIPEDIA

WEBSITE: www.wikipedia.org

Often maligned because "anybody" can start an entry or edit an existing entry, Wikipedia is the largest repository of general information on every conceivable subject on planet Earth. It is an enormous encyclopedia and while some entries on the subject of nutrients are rather limited and also include a lot of talk about the molecular structures and methods of synthesis, it is still one of the best online resources that covers all subjects and each page does include the references which you can pursue as well. Whenever they ask for a few dollars, please give, so we can keep this vast repository of information free and unencumbered by advertising.

"SUPERFOODLY"

WEBSITE ADDRESS: www.superfoodly.com

This site covers a lot of ground and lists the ORAC – Oxygen Radical Absorption Capacity – scores for hundreds of different foods, mostly natural whole foods. I highly recommend this website as a way to "shop for" new antioxidant-rich foods to add to your own natural whole foods diet.

NUTRITION DATA at SELF.COM

WEBSITE: http://nutritiondata.self.com

This is one of the largest repositories of detailed nutrient analyses of a wide range of foods, both packaged as well as natural whole foods, imaginable. The original source of the data is the FDA website, but this website has it in a far better format. You can search for many natural whole foods and they will most likely have the complete nutrition label including every vitamin, mineral, and many other nutrients as well as "undesirable" constituents listed in that label including cholesterol, saturated fat and the sugars and starches (the "Carb Load".) Unfortunately, those labels do not include Molybdenum and Iodine (both covered at the George Mateljan Foundation's website) but the total information provided for each food is still very useful.

"WEB MD"

WEBSITE ADDRESS: www.webmd.com

Aside from having an extensive collection of articles on the nutrients, WebMD also includes many articles on prevention and treatment for just about every ailment as well.

SOURCES OF DIETARY/HERBAL SUPPLEMENTS

I have not been able to check into most of these manufacturers because there are literally many hundreds of them. You will have to verify the quality and authenticity of their products by searching for neutral third party reviews of their products (such as Consumer Reports.)

GARDEN of LIFE – www.gardenoflife.com – This company makes a whole line of supplements based on natural extract sources of very high quality; many of their products have no competition that I could find: no other natural extract product of the same nutrient(s) on the market, just synthetics. Some of their products are never exposed to temperatures above 115°F which would destroy many nutrients during manufacture. The products are not inexpensive but they are definitely the very best that I could find.

JARROW FORMULAS – www.jarrow.com – This is another manufacturer of very high quality dietary supplements.

NOW FOODS – www.nowfoods.com – An excellent high quality dietary supplement manufacturer.

PURITANS PRIDE – www.puritanspride.com – This vendor also carries many different natural whole food products and supplements as well as their own.

SWANSON VITAMINS – www.swansonvitamins.com – While they do carry many other brands, this company makes a lot of holistic herbal supplements, many of which can't be found anywhere else.

VITACOST – www.vitacost.com – This is a large online dietary supplement and natural foods vendor. They carry hundreds of brands and also manufacture some very high quality products under their own brand name labels.

BULK HOLISTIC HERBS

There aren't many vendors that sell plain bulk dried medicinal herbs, but in the long run the cost is better although you would have to prepare your own herbal teas rather than buy prepared prepackaged herbal supplements.

MOUNTAIN ROSE HERBS – www.mountainroseherbs.com – These people have an impressive inventory of holistic herbs available in bulk packages, essential oils, or seeds for those who want to grow their own.

BULK APOTHECARY – www.bulkapothecary.com Included because they do have a selection of holistic herbal bulk products.

I have included the following websites because they each have at least one product that no one else carries.

TRADITIONAL MEDICINALS – www.traditionalmedicinals.com

HERB Co. – www.herbco.com/c-2-bulk-herbs-spices.aspx

STAR WEST BOTANICALS – www.starwest-botanicals.com/category/bulk-organic-herbs/

FRONTIER COOP – www.frontiercoop.com/bulk-products/herbs/

HERB AFFAIR – www.herbaffair.com/collections/herbs-and-spices

REFERENCES

[1] Vitamin A: https://draxe.com/top-10-vitamin-foods/ Retrieved 7/23/18 *
https://www.myfooddata.com/articles/food-sources-of-vitamin-A.php
Retrieved 7/23/18 * http://www.whfoods.com/genpage.php?tname=
nutrient&dbid=106 Retrieved 7/23/18

[2] Vitamin B1 - Thiamine: https://draxe.com/thiamine-foods/ Retrieved
7/23/18

[3] Vitamin B2 - Riboflavin: * https://draxe.com/vitamin-b2/ Retrieved
7/23/18 * https://www.myfooddata.com/articles/foods-high-in-
riboflavin-vitamin-B2.php Retrieved 7/23/18 * www.whfoods.com/
genpage.php?tname=nutrient&dbid=93 Retrieved 7/23/18

[4] Vitamin B3 - Niacin: * https://draxe.com/niacin-side-effects/ Retrieved
7/24/18 * https://www.myfooddata.com/articles/foods-high-in-niacin-
vitamin-B3.php Retrieved 7/24/18 * www.whfoods.com/genpage.php
?tname=nutrient&dbid=83 Retrieved 7/24/18

[5] Vitamin B5 – Pantothenic acid: * https://draxe.com/vitamin-b5/
Retrieved 7/24/18 * http://www.whfoods.com/genpage.php?tname
=nutrient&dbid=87 Retrieved 7/24/18 * https://en.wikipedia.org/wiki/
Pantothenic_acid Retrieved 7/24/18

[6] Vitamin B6 - Pyridoxine: * https://draxe.com/top-10-vitamin-b6-foods/
Retrieved 7/24/18 * http://www.whfoods.com/genpage.php?tname\
=nutrient&dbid=108 Retrieved 7/24/18

[7] Vitamin B7 - Biotin: * https://draxe.com/biotin-benefits/ Retrieved
7/24/18 * https://en.wikipedia.org/wiki/Biotin Retrieved 7/24/18

[8] Vitamin B9 – Folic acid: * https://draxe.com/top-10-vitamin-b9-folate-
foods/ Retrieved 7/24/18 * http://www.whfoods.com/genpage.php?
tname=nutrient&dbid=63 Retrieved 7/24/18

[9] Vitamin B12 - Methylcobalamin: https://draxe.com/vitamin-b12-benefits/
Retrieved 7/24/18 * https://en.wikipedia.org/wiki/Cobalamin Retrieved
7/24/18

[10] Choline: * https://draxe.com/what-is-choline/ Retrieved 7/24/18 *
http://www.whfoods.com/genpage.php?tname=nutrient&dbid=50
Retrieved 7/24/18

[11] Vitamin C: * https://draxe.com/vitamin-c-benefits/ Retrieved 7/26/18 *
https://www.myfooddata.com/articles/vitamin-c-foods.php Retrieved
7/26/18 * http://www.whfoods.com/genpage.php?tname=nutrient
&dbid=109 Retrieved 7/26/18

[12] Vitamin D3 – Cholecalciferol: https://draxe.com/vitamin-d-deficiency-
symptoms/ Retrieved 7/26/18 * https://www.myfooddata.com/
articles/high-vitamin-D-foods.php Retrieved 7/26/18 *
http://www.whfoods.com/genpage.php?tname=nutrient&dbid=110
Retrieved 7/26/18

[13] Vitamin E – alpha-Tocopherol: * https://draxe.com/vitamin-e-foods/
Retrieved 7/26/18 * https://www.myfooddata.com/articles/vitamin-e-
foods.php Retrieved 7/26/18 * http://www.whfoods.com/genpage.php
?tname=nutrient&dbid=111 Retrieved 7/26/18

[14] Vitamin K – n-Quinones: https://draxe.com/vitamin-k-deficiency/
Retrieved 7/26/18 * https://www.myfooddata.com/articles/food-
sources-of-vitamin-k.php Retrieved 7/26/18 * www.whfoods.com/
genpage.php?tname=nutrient&dbid=112 Retrieved 7/26/18

[15] Calcium: https://draxe.com/foods-high-in-calcium/ Retrieved 7/30/18 *
https://www.myfooddata.com/articles/foods-high-in-calcium.php
Retrieved 7/30/18 * http://www.whfoods.com/genpage.php?tname
=nutrient&dbid=45 Retrieved 7/30/18

[16] Chlorine: www.quora.com/Does-the-body-need-chlorine Retrieved 01-03-2019

[17] Chromium: https://draxe.com/what-is-chromium/ Retrieved 8/23/18 * http://www.whfoods.com/genpage.php?tname=nutrient&dbid=51 Retrieved 8/23/18

[18] Copper: https://draxe.com/foods-high-in-copper/ Retrieved 8/23/18 * https://www.myfooddata.com/articles/high-copper-foods.php Retrieved 8/23/18 * http://www.whfoods.com/genpage.php?tname=nutrient&dbid=53 Retrieved 8/23/18

[19] Iodine: https://draxe.com/iodine-rich-foods/ Retrieved 7/26/18 * https://www.myfooddata.com/articles/natural-foods-high-in-iodine.php Retrieved 7/26/18

[20] Iron: * https://draxe.com/top-10-iron-rich-foods/ Retrieved 7/30/18 * https://www.myfooddata.com/articles/food-sources-of-iron.php Retrieved 7/30/18 * http://www.whfoods.com/genpage.php?tname=nutrient&dbid=70 Retrieved 7/30/18

[21] Magnesium: https://draxe.com/magnesium-deficient-top-10-magnesium-rich-foods-must-eating/ Retrieved 7/30/18 * https://www.myfooddata.com/articles/foods-high-in-magnesium.php Retrieved 7/30/18 * http://www.whfoods.com/genpage.php?tname=nutrient&dbid=75 Retrieved 7/30/18

[22] Manganese: https://draxe.com/manganese/ Retrieved 8/23/18 * https://www.myfooddata.com/articles/foods-high-in-manganese.php Retrieved 8/23/18

[23] Molybdenum: http://www.whfoods.com/genpage.php?tname=nutrient&dbid=128 Retrieved 8/29/18

[24] Phosphorus: https://draxe.com/foods-high-in-phosphorus/ Retrieved 7/30/18 * https://www.myfooddata.com/articles/high-phosphorus-foods.php Retrieved 7/30/18 * http://www.whfoods.com/genpage.php?tname=nutrient&dbid=127 Retrieved 7/30/18

[25] Potassium: https://draxe.com/low-potassium/ Retrieved 8/23/18 * https://www.myfooddata.com/articles/food-sources-of-potassium.php Retrieved 8/23/18

[26] Selenium: https://draxe.com/selenium-foods/ Retrieved 8/23/18 * https://www.myfooddata.com/articles/foods-high-in-selenium.php Retrieved 8/23/18 * http://www.whfoods.com/genpage.php?tname=nutrient&dbid=95 Retrieved 8/23/18

[27] Sodium: https://draxe.com/low-potassium/ Retrieved 8/23/18

[28] Sulfur: https://articles.mercola.com/sites/articles/archive/2016/05/16/sulfur-in-the-body.aspx Retreived on 01-03-2019

[29] Zinc: https://draxe.com/foods-high-in-zinc/ Retrieved 8/23/18 * https://www.myfooddata.com/articles/high-zinc-foods.php Retrieved 8/23/18 * http://www.whfoods.com/genpage.php?tname=nutrient&dbid=115 Retrieved 8/23/18

[30] Walnuts: https://nutritiondata.self.com/facts/nut-and-seed-products/3138/2 Retrieved 9/12/18

[31] Almonds: https://nutritiondata.self.com/facts/nut-and-seed-products/3087/2 Retrieved 9/12/18

[32] Sunflower seed kernels: https://nutritiondata.self.com/facts/nut-and-seed-products/3077/2 Retrieved 9/12/18

[33] Peanuts and peanut butter: https://nutritiondata.self.com/facts/legumes-and-legume-products/4453/2 Retrieved 9/12/18

[34] Antioxidants: https://draxe.com/top-10-high-antioxidant-foods/ Retrieved 8/20/18 * http://www.superfoodly.com (ORAC scores)

Retrieved 8/29/18

[35] Kiwi: https://nutritiondata.self.com/facts/fruits-and-fruit-juices/1934/2 Retrieved 9/12/18

[36] Grapefruit: https://nutritiondata.self.com/facts/fruits-and-fruit-juices/1905/2 Retrieved 9/12/18 * www.anniesremedy.com/citrus-paradisi-grapefruit.php Retrieved 12/20/18 * www.stuartxchange.org/Suha.html Retrieved 12/5/18

[37] Cabbage: https://nutritiondata.self.com/facts/vegetables-and-vegetable-products/2372/2 Retrieved 9/12/18 * www.stuartxchange.org/Repolyo.html Retrieved 12/5/18

[38] Carrots: https://nutritiondata.self.com/facts/vegetables-and-vegetable-products/2383/2 Retrieved 9/12/18 * www.stuartxchange.org/Karot.html Retrieved 12/5/18

[39] Bearberry: www.anniesremedy.com/arctostaphylos-uva-ursi.php Retrieved 12/20/18

[40] Black Pepper: www.anniesremedy.com/piper-nigrum-black-pepper.php Retrieved 12/20/18

[41] Buchu: www.anniesremedy.com/agathosma-betulina.php Retrieved 12/20/18

[42] Salmon: https://nutritiondata.self.com/facts/ethnic-foods/10460/2 Retrieved 9/12/18

[43] Wheat germ: https://nutritiondata.self.com/facts/cereal-grains-and-pasta/5743/2 Retrieved 9/12/18

[44] Parmesan (and Romano) cheese: https://nutritiondata.self.com/facts/dairy-and-egg-products/32/2 Retrieved 9/12/18

[45] Swiss cheese: https://nutritiondata.self.com/facts/dairy-and-egg-products/39/2 Retrieved 9/12/18

[46] Yogurt: https://nutritiondata.self.com/facts/dairy-and-egg-products/104/2 Retrieved 9/12/18

[47] Cod Liver Oil: https://nutritiondata.self.com/facts/fats-and-oils/628/2 Retrieved 9/12/18

[48] Beef liver: https://nutritiondata.self.com/facts/beef-products/3468/2 Retrieved 9/12/18

[49] Broccoli: https://nutritiondata.self.com/facts/vegetables-and-vegetable-products/2356/2 Retrieved 9/12/18

[50] Grapes, grape seed, and grape juice: https://draxe.com/grapes-nutrition/ Retrieved 9/12/18 * www.anniesremedy.com/vitis-vinifera-grapes.php Retrieved 12/20/18

[51] Jaboticaba: www.stuartxchange.org/Jaboticaba.html Retrieved 12/5/18

[52] The 9 Essential Amino Acids: * https://bareblends.com.au/blog/the-9-essential-amino-acids-what-are-they-and-why-do-we-need-them/ Retrieved 8/23/18 * http://en.wikipedia.org/Essential_amino_acid Retrieved 3/26/19

[53] Oysters: https://nutritiondata.self.com/facts/finfish-and-shellfish-products/4192/2 Retrieved 9/12/18

[54] Clams: https://nutritiondata.self.com/facts/finfish-and-shellfish-products/4183/2 Retrieved 9/12/18

[55] Pumpkin Seeds: https://nutritiondata.self.com/facts/nut-and-seed-products/3141/2 Retrieved 9/12/18

[56] Pistachios: https://nutritiondata.self.com/facts/nut-and-seed-products/3136/2 Retrieved 9/12/18 * http://draxe.com/foods-lower-blood-pressure.html Retrieved 9/10/18

[57] Dark chocolate: https://nutritiondata.self.com/facts/sweets/5390/2 Retrieved 9/12/18 * www.anniesremedy.com/theobroma-cacao.php

Retrieved 12/20/18 * www.stuartxchange.org/Kakaw.html Retrieved 12/5/18

[58] Spirulina: https://nutritiondata.self.com/facts/vegetables-and-vegetable-products/2765/2 Retrieved 9/12/18

[59] Omega-3 Fatty Acids: https://draxe.com/omega-3-benefits-plus-top-10-omega-3-foods-list/ Retrieved 8/23/18 * www.myfooddata.com/articles/high-omega-3-foods.php Retrieved 8/23/18

[60] Atlantic Mackerel: https://nutritiondata.self.com/facts/finfish-and-shellfish-products/4072/2 Retrieved 9/12/18

[61] Tuna: https://nutritiondata.self.com/facts/finfish-and-shellfish-products/4206/2 Retrieved 9/12/18

[62] Sardines: https://nutritiondata.self.com/facts/finfish-and-shellfish-products/4114/2 Retrieved 9/12/18

[63] Chickpeas: https://nutritiondata.self.com/facts/legumes-and-legume-products/4325/2 Retrieved 9/12/18

[64] Lentils: https://nutritiondata.self.com/facts/legumes-and-legume-products/4337/2 Retrieved 9/12/18

[65] Brazil nuts: https://nutritiondata.self.com/facts/nut-and-seed-products/3091/2 Retrieved 9/12/18

[66] Spinach: https://nutritiondata.self.com/facts/vegetables-and-vegetable-products/2626/2 Retrieved 9/12/18 * www.stuartxchange.org/Spinach.html Retrieved 12/5/18

[67] Kale: https://nutritiondata.self.com/facts/vegetables-and-vegetable-products/2461/2 Retrieved 9/12/18

[68] Oats: https://nutritiondata.self.com/facts/breakfast-cereals/1597/2 Retrieved 9/12/18 * www.anniesremedy.com/avena-sativa-oats.php Retrieved 12/20/18

[69] Banana: https://nutritiondata.self.com/facts/fruits-and-fruit-juices/1846/2 Retrieved 9/12/18 * www.stuartxchange.org/Saging.html Retrieved 12/5/18

[70] Green peas: https://nutritiondata.self.com/facts/vegetables-and-vegetable-products/2888/2 Retrieved 9/12/18

[71] Omega-6 fatty acids: https://draxe.com/omega-6/ Retrieved 8/20/18

[72] Swiss cheese: https://nutritiondata.self.com/facts/dairy-and-egg-products/39/2 Retrieved 9/12/18

[73] Low Sodium V-8: https://nutritiondata.self.com/facts/vegetables-and-vegetable-products/10452/2 Retrieved 9/12/18

[74] Lamb: https://nutritiondata.self.com/facts/lamb-veal-and-game-products/4474/2 Retrieved 9/12/18

[75] Ashwagandha: https://www.anniesremedy.com/withania-somnifera-ashwagandha-root.php Retrieved 12/20/18

[76] Cranberry: https://www.anniesremedy.com/vaccinium-macrocarpon-cranberry.php Retrieved 12/20/18

[77] Cumin: https://www.anniesremedy.com/cuminum-cyminum.php Retrieved 12/20/18

[78] Dandelion: www.anniesremedy.com/taraxacum-officinale-dandelion-root.php Retrieved 12/20/18

[79] Horsetail: www.anniesremedy.com/equisetum-arvense-horsetail.php Retrieved 12/20/18

[80] Butcher's Broom: https://www.anniesremedy.com/ruscus-aculeatus-butcher-broom.php Retrieved 12/20/18

[81] Celery: www.anniesremedy.com/apium-graviolens-celery-seed.php Retrieved 12/20/18 * www.stuartxchange.org/Kintsay.html

[82] Cleavers: www.anniesremedy.com/galium-aparine-cleavers.php Retrieved 12/20/18

[83] Chanca Piedra: www.anniesremedy.com/phyllanthus-niruri-chanca-piedra.php Retrieved 12/20/18 * ww.stuartxchange.org/Ibaibaan.html Retrieved 12/5/18

[84] Juniper: www.anniesremedy.com/juniperus-communis-juniper-berries.php Retrieved 12/20/18

[85] Lavender: www.anniesremedy.com/lavandula-spp.php Retrieved 12/20/18 * www.stuartxchange.org/Lavandula.html Retrieved 12/5/18

[86] Cinnamon: www.anniesremedy.com/cinnamomum-zeylanicum-cinnamon.php Retrieved 12/20/18 * www.stuartxchange.org/Kalingag.html Retrieved 12/5/18

[87] Lovage: www.anniesremedy.com/levisticum-officinale-lovage.php Retrieved 12/20/18

[88] Coleus: www.anniesremedy.com/plectranthus-barbatus-coleus-forskohlii php Retrieved 12/20/18

[89] Coriander: www.anniesremedy.com/coriandrum-sativum-coriander.php Retrieved 12/20/18 * www.stuartxchange.org/Kulantro.html Retrieved 12/5/18

[90] Motherwort: www.anniesremedy.com/leonurus-cardica-motherwort.php Retrieved 12/20/18

[91] Parsley: www.anniesremedy.com/petroselinum-crispum-parsley.php Retrieved 12/20/18

[92] Plantain: www.anniesremedy.com/plantago-major-lanceolata-plantain.php Retrieved 12/20/18

[93] Rehmannia: www.anniesremedy.com/rehmannia-glutinosa-rehmannia-root.php Retrieved 12/20/18

[94] Rosemary: www.anniesremedy.com/rosmarinus-officinalis-rosemary.php Retrieved 12/20/18 * www.stuartxchange.org/Romero.html Retrieved 12/5/18

[95] Stinging Nettle: www.anniesremedy.com/urtica-dioica-stinging-nettle.php Retrieved 12/20/18

[96] Fever Bark: www.stuartxchange.org/Dita.html Retrieved 12/5/18

[97] Watercress: https:/nutritiondata.self.com/facts/vegetables-and-vegetable-products/2718/2 Retrieved 3/18/19 * www.anniesremedy.com/nasturtium-officinale-watercress.php Retrieved 12/20/18 * http://whfoods.com/genpage.php?tname =foodspice&dbid=31 Retrieved 3/19/19

[98] Açai: www.anniesremedy.com/euterpe-oleracea-acai-berry.php Retrieved 12/20/18

[99] Garlic: www.anniesremedy.com/allium-sativum-garlic.php Retrieved 12/20/18 * www.stuartxchange.org/Bawang.html * Garlic: https://www.webmd.com/vitamins/ai/ingredientmono-300/garlic Retrieved 9/18/18

[100] Bitter Melon: www.anniesremedy.com/momordica-charantia-bitter-melon.php Retrieved 12/20/18

[101] Banaba: www.stuartxchange.org/Banaba.html Retrieved 12/5/18

[102] Hibiscus: www.anniesremedy.com/hibiscus-sabdariffa-hibiscus-tea.php Retrieved 12/20/18 * www.stuartxchange.org/Gumamela.html Retrieved 12/5/18

[103] Hog Weed: www.stuartxchange.org/Paanbalibis.html Retrieved 12/5/18

[104] Coconut: www.anniesremedy.com/cocos-nucifera-coconut-oil.php Retrieved 12/20/18 * www.stuartxchange.org/Niyog2.html Retrieved

12/5/18

[105] Hyssop: www.anniesremedy.com/hyssopus-officinalis-hyssop.php Retrieved 12/20/18 * www.stuartxchange.org/Hyssop.html Retrieved 12/5/18

[106] Jiaogulan: www.anniesremedy.com/gynostemma-pentaphyllum-jiaogulan.php Retrieved 12/20/18

[107] Job's Tears: www.stuartxchange.org/Katigbi.html Retrieved 12/5/18

[108] Coffee: www.anniesremedy.com/coffea-arabica.php Retrieved 12/20/18

[109] Guarana: www.anniesremedy.com/paullinia-cupana-guarana.php Retrieved 12/20/18

[110] Licorice: www.anniesremedy.com/glycyrrhiza-glabra-licorice-root.php Retrieved 12/20/18

[111] Lemon/Lime: www.anniesremedy.com/citrus-aurantifolia-lime-oil.php Retrieved 12/20/18 * www.anniesremedy.com/citrus-liminum-lemon.php Retrieved 12/20/18 * www.stuartxchange.org/Dayap.html Retrieved 12/5/18

[112] Lotus: www.anniesremedy.com/nelumbo-nucifera-lotus.php Retrieved 12/20/18 * www.stuartxchange.org/Baino.html Retrieved 12/5/18

[113] Marjoram: www.anniesremedy.com/origanum-majorana-marjoram-sweet.php Retrieved 12/20/18 * www.stuartxchange.org/Marjoram.html Retrieved 12/5/18

[114] Olives: http://draxe.com/foods-lower-blood-pressure.html Retrieved 9/10/18

[115] Maitake Mushroom: www.anniesremedy.com/grifola-frondosa-maitake-mushroom.php Retrieved 12/20/18

[116] Nut grass: www.stuartxchange.org/Mutha.html Retrieved 12/5/18

[117] Tea: www.stuartxchange.org/Tsa.html Retrieved 12/5/18

[118] Acerola: www.stuartxchange.org/Acerola.html Retrieved 12/5/18 * https://nutritiondata.self.com/facts/fruits-and-fruit-juices/1807/2

[119] Chickweed: www.anniesremedy.com/stellaria-media-chickweed.php Retrieved 12/20/18

[120] Dates: www.stuartxchange.org/DatePalm.html Retrieved 12/5/18

[121] Fennel: www.anniesremedy.com/foeniculum-vulgare-fennel-seed.php Retrieved 12/20/18

[122] Gamboge: www.anniesremedy.com/garcinia-cambogia-fruit.php Retrieved 12/20/18

[123] Gurmar: www.anniesremedy.com/gtmnema-sylvestre-gurmar.php Retrieved 12/20/18

[124] Heavenly elixir: www.stuartxchange.org/Makabuhay.html Retrieved 12/5/18

[125] Hoodia: www.anniesremedy.com/hoodia-gordonii.php Retrieved 12/20/18

[126] Jew's mallow: www.stuartxchange.org/Pasau.html Retrieved 12/5/18

[127] Jujube: www.stuartxchange.org/Mansanitas.html Retrieved 12/5/18

[128] Lima beans: www.stuartxchange.org/Patani.html Retrieved 12/5/18

[129] New Zealand spinach: www.stuartxchange.org/Sabungai.html Retrieved 12/5/18

[130] Onion: www.stuartxchange.org/Sibuyas.html Retrieved 12/5/18

[131] Prickly Pear: www.anniesremedy.com/opuntia-ficus-indica-prickly-pear.php Retrieved 12/20/18

[132] Psyllium: www.anniesremedy.com/plantago-psyllium-ovata.php Retrieved 12/20/18

[133] Safflower Oil (CLA): www.anniesremedy.com/carthamis-tinctorius-safflower-oil.php Retrieved 12/20/18

[134] Sage: www.anniesremedy.com/salvia-officinalis-sage.php Retrieved 12/20/18

[135] Smartweed: www.stuartxchange.org/Buding.html Retrieved 12/5/18

[136] Star Fruit: www.stuartxchange.org/Balimbing.html Retrieved 12/5/18

[137] Stevia: www.anniesremedy.com/stecia-rebaudiana.php Retrieved 12/20/18 [139]

[138] Sugar cane: www.stuartxchange.org/Tubo.html Retrieved 12/5/18

[139] Tamarind: www.stuartxchange.org/Sampalok.html Retrieved 12/5/18

[140] Winged treebine: www.stuartxchange.org/Sugpon-sugpon.html

[141] Yerba mate: www.anniesremedy.com/ilex-paraguariensis-yerba-mate.php Retrieved 12/20/18

[142] Astragalus: www.anniesremedy.com/astragalus-membranaceus-root.php Retrieved 12/20/18

[143] Cut-leaved Panax: www.stuartxchange.org/Papua.html Retrieved 12/5/18

[144] Flax Seed: www.anniesremedy.com/linum-usitatissimum-flax-seed.php Retrieved 12/20/18

[145] Chia seed: http://draxe.com/foods-lower-blood-pressure.html Retrieved 9/10/18 * www.stuartxchange.org/Chia.html Retrieved 12/5/18

[146] Dong Quai: www.anniesremedy.com/angelica-sinensis-dong-quai.php Retrieved 12/20/18

[147] Electric Daisy: www.stuartxchange.org/Biri.html Retrieved 12/5/18

[148] Eleuthero: www.anniesremedy.com/eleuterococcus-senticosus-eleuthero-root.php Retrieved 12/20/18

[149] Fo-ti: www.anniesremedy.com/polygonum-multiflorum-fo-ti-root.php Retrieved 12/20/18

[150] Ginger: www.anniesremedy.com/zingiber-officinale-ginger-root.php Retrieved 12/20/18 * www.stuartxchange.org/Luya.html Retrieved 12/5/18

[151] Ginseng (Asian): www.anniesremedy.com/panax-ginseng-root.php Retrieved 12/20/18

[152] Hog Plum: www.stuartxchange.org/Libas.html Retrieved 12/5/18

[153] Holy Basil: www.anniesremedy.com/ocimum-sanctum-holy-basil.php Retrieved 12/20/18 * www.stuartxchange.org/Sulasi.html Retrieved 12/5/18

[154] Maca: www.anniesremedy.com/lepidium-peruvianum-maca-rootl.php Retrieved 12/20/18

[155] Peppermint: www.anniesremedy.com/mentha-piperita-peppermint.php Retrieved 12/20/18 * www.stuartxchange.org/Yerba.html Retrieved 12/5/18

[156] Rhodiola: www.anniesremedy.com/rhodiola-rosea-rhodiola.php Retrieved 12/20/18

[157] Schisandra: www.anniesremedy.com/schisandra-chinensis.php Retrieved 12/20/18

[158] Suma Root: www.anniesremedy.com/pfaffia-paniculata-suma-root.php Retrieved 12/20/18

[159] Butternut Squash: www.draxe.com/butternut-squash-nutrition/ Retrieved 3/16/19 * https://nutritiondata.self.com/facts/vegetables-and-vegetable-products/2647/2 Retrieved 3/8/19

[160] Sweet Potatoes: https://nutritiondata.self.com/facts/vegetables-and-vegetable-products/2667/2 Retrieved 3/8/19

[161] Yeast Extract Spread: https://nutritiondata.self.com/facts/vegetables-and-vebetable-products/7691/2 Retrieved 3/19/19

{162} Pork (chops): https://nutritiondata.self.com/facts/pork-products/2155/2 Retrieved 3/18/19

[163] Button Mushrooms: http://whfoods.com/genpage.php?tname=foodspice&dbid=97 Retrieved 3/8/19 *

[164] Chicken: https://nutritiondata.self.com/facts/poultry-products/701/2 Retrieved 3/16/13

[165] Chicken Liver: https://nutritiondata.self.com/facts/poultry-products/666/2 Retrieved 3/16/13

[166] Beef (Sirloin): https://nutritiondata.self.com/facts/beef-products/3591/2 Retrieved 3/8/19

[167] Annual Mortality Statistics – Centers for Disease Control: https://www.cdc.gov/nchs/fastats/deaths.htm

[168] Cauliflower: http://whfoods.com/genpage.php?tname=foodspice&dbid=13 Retrieved 3/8/19

[169] Turnip greens: https://nutritiondata.self.com/facts/vegetables-and-vegetable-products/7680/2 Retrieved 5/20/19

[170] Bok Choy: http://whfoods.com/genpage.php?tname=foodspice&dbid=152Retrieved 3/8/19

[171] Bell Pepper: http://whfoods.com/genpage.php?tname=foodspice&dbid=50 Retrieved 3/8/19

[172] Okra: https://nutritiondata.self.com/facts/vegetables-and/vegetable-products/2497/2 Retrieved 3/16/19 * https://articles.mercola.com/sites/articles/archive/2016/08/15/health-benefits-of-okra.aspx Retrieved 3/8/19

[173] Tomato: www.stuartxchange.org/Kamatis.html Retrieved 12/5/18 * http://whfoods.com/genpage.php?tname=foodspice&dbid=44 Retrieved 3/19/19

[174] Asparagus: http://whfoods.com/genpage.php?tname=foodspice&dbid=3 Retrieved 3/8/19

[175] Scallops: http://www.whfoods.com/genpage.php?tname=nutrientprofile&dbid=105 Retrieved 3/16/19

[176] Guava: www.stuartxchange.org/Bayabas.html Retrieved 12/5/18 * https://nutritiondata.self.com/facts/fruits-and-fruit-juices/1927/2 Retrieved 3/8/19

[177] Milk: https://nutritiondata.self.com/facts/dairy-and-egg-products/69/2 Retrieved 3/8/19

[178] Swiss Chard: http://whfoods.com/genpage.php?tname=foodspice&dbid=16 Retrieved 3/19/19

[179] Collard Greens: https://nutritiondata.self.com/facts/vegetables-and-vegetable-products/2411/2 Retrieved 3/8/19

[180] Black Plums and Dried Plums: https://nutritiondata.self.com/facts/fruits-and-fruit-juices/2043/2 and https://nutritiondata.self.com/facts/fruits-and-fruit-juices/2032/2 Retrieved 4/6/19 * http://whfoods.com/genpage.php?tname=foodspice &dbid=35 Retrieved 3/19/19

[181] Eggs: https://nutritiondata.self.com/facts/dairy-and-egg-products/117/2 Retrieved 3/8/19

[182] Brussels Sprouts: http://whfoods.com/genpage.php?tname=foodspice&dbid=10 Retrieved 3/8/19

[183] Beets: http://whfoods.com/genpage.php?tname=foodspice&dbid=49 Retrieved 3/8/19

[184] Pumpkin: https://nutritiondata.self.com/facts/vegetables-and/vegetable-products/2602/2 Retrieved 3/16/19

[185] Mussels: https://nutritiondata.self.com/facts/finfish-and-shellfish-products/4187/2 Retrieved 3/8/19

[186] Pollock: https://nutritiondata.self.com/facts/finfish-and-shellfish-products/4091/2 Retrieved 12/5/18

[187] Napa Cabbage: https://nutritiondata.self.com/facts/vegetables-and-vegetable-products/3035/2 Retrieved 3/16/19

[188] Green Beans: https://nutritiondata.self.com/facts/vegetables-and-vebetable-products/2805/2 Retrieved 3/19/19

[189] Pineapple: http://whfoods.com/genpage.php?tname=foodspice&dbid=34 Retrieved 3/8/19

[190] Black Beans: https://nutritiondata.self.com/facts/legumes-and-legume-products/4287/2 Retrieved 3/8/19 * http://whfoods.com/genpage.php?tname=foodspice&dbid=2 Retrieved 3/8/19

[191] Cucumber: http://whfoods.com/genpage.php?tname=foodspice&dbid=42 Retrieved 3/8/19

[192] Shrimp: http://whfoods.com/genpage.php?tname=foodspice&dbid=107 Retrieved 3/8/19

[193] Cod: https://nutritiondata.self.com/facts/finfish-and-shellfish-products/4041/2 Retrieved 3/9/13

[194] Zucchini: https://nutritiondata.self.com/facts/vegetables-and-vegetable-products/2640/2 Retrieved 3/16/19

[195] Yams: https://foodfacts.mercola.com/yam.html Retrieved 3/18/19 * https://nutritiondata.self.com/facts/vegetables-and-vegetable-products/2726/2 Retrieved 3/18/19

[196] Turkey: https://nutritiondata.self.com/facts/poultry-products/825/2 Retrieved 3/16/13

[197] Veal: https://nutritiondata.self.com/facts/lamb-veal-and-game-products/4747/2 Retrieved 3/16/19

[198] Venison: https://nutritiondata.self.com/facts/lamb-veal-and-game-products/4814/2 Retrieved 4/1/19

[199] Goat: https://nutritiondata.self.com/facts/lamb-veal-and-game-products/4637/2 * Retrieved 4/6/19

[200] Ham (deli): https://nutritiondata.self.com/facts/sausages-and-luncheon-meats/1345/2 Retrieved 3/18/19

[201] Fava Beans: https://nutritiondata.self.com/facts/legumes-and-legume-products/4323/2 Retrieved 3/16/19

[202] Blackeye Peas: https://nutritiondata.self.com/facts/legumes-and-legume-products/4333/2 Retrieved 3/8/19

[203] Avocado: http://whfoods.com/genpage.php?tname=foodspice&dbid=5 Retrieved 3/8/19 * www.stuartxchange.org/Abukado.html Retrieved 12/5/18

[204] Pecans: https://nutritiondata.self.com/facts/nut-and-seed-products/3130/2 Retrieved 3/8/19

[205] Fiber: http://draxe.com/high-fiber-foods Retrieved on 8/13/18 * http://www.whfoods.com/genpage.php?tname=nutrient&dbid=128 Retrieved 8/29/18

[206] Cut-leaved Panax: www.stuartxchange.org/Papua.html Retrieved 12/5/18

[207] Rooibos: https://www.anniesremedy.com/aspalathus-linearis-rooibos.php Retrieved 12/20/18

[208] Tangerine: https://nutritiondata.self.com/facts/fruits-and-fruit-juices/1978/2 Retrieved 3/8/19 * https://drhealthbenefits.com/food-bevarages/fruits/health-benefits-of-tangerines

[209] Avocado: http://whfoods.com/genpage.php?tname=foodspice

&dbid=5 Retrieved 3/8/19 * www.stuartxchange.org/Abukado.html Retrieved 12/5/18

[210] Cantaloupe: http://whfoods.com/genpage.php?tname=foodspice &dbid=17 Retrieved 3/8/19

[211] Dates: www.stuartxchange.org/DatePalm.html Retrieved 12/5/18

[212] Dragon Fruit: www.stuartxchange.org/DragonFruit.html Retrieved 12/5/18

[213] Gardenia: www.stuartxchange.org/Rosal.html Retrieved 12/5/18

[214] Kelp: Edwards, Rebekah, https://draxe.com/kelp/ Retrieved 4/16/19 * https://nutritiondata.self.com/facts/vegetables-and-vegetable-products/2617/2 Retrieved 3/8/19

[215] Mangosteen: www.stuartxchange.org/Mangosteen.html Retrieved 12/5/18

[216] Oregano: www.stuartxchange.org/Oregano.html Retrieved 12/5/18 * www.anniesremedy.com/origanum-vulgare-oregano.php Retrieved 12/20/18

[217] Turmeric: www.anniesremedy.com/curcuma-longa-turmeric.php Retrieved 12/20/18 * www.stuartxchange.org/Dilaw.html Retrieved 12/5/18

[218] Wild Almond: www.stuartxchange.org/Kalumpang.html Retrieved 12/5/18